Second Edition

The Real ABCs

ACHIEVEMENT, BALANCE, CONTENTMENT

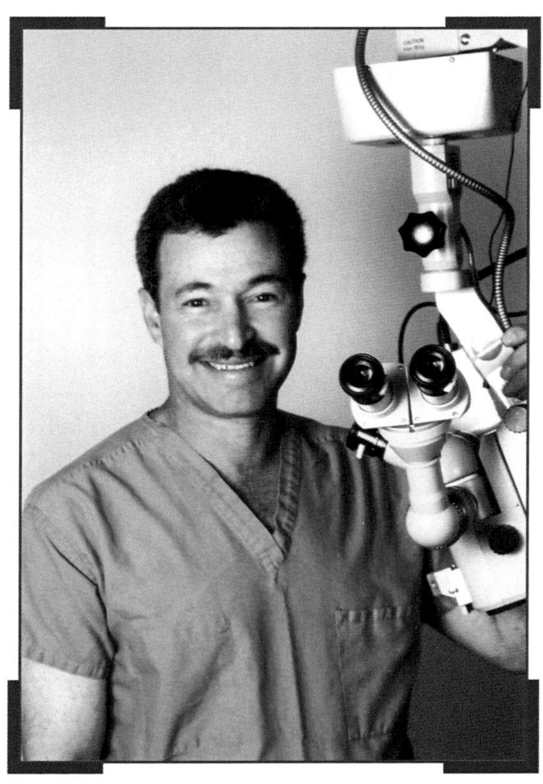

Second Edition

The Real ABCs

ACHIEVEMENT, BALANCE, CONTENTMENT

Robert H. Osher, MD
Professor of Ophthalmology
University of Cincinnati College of Medicine
Medical Director Emeritus
Cincinnati Eye Institute
Cincinnati, Ohio
Founder and Editor
Video Journal of Cataract, Refractive, & Glaucoma Surgery

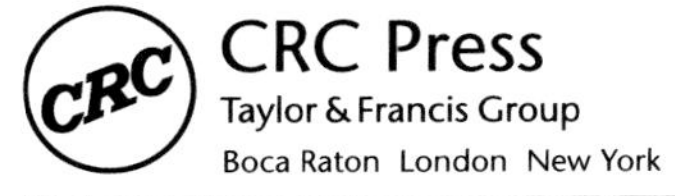

CRC Press
Taylor & Francis Group
Boca Raton London New York

CRC Press is an imprint of the
Taylor & Francis Group, an **informa** business

Dr. Robert H. Osher has no financial or proprietary interest in the materials presented herein.

First published 2020 by SLACK Incorporated

Published 2024 by CRC Press
2385 NW Executive Center Drive, Suite 320, Boca Raton FL 33431

and by CRC Press
4 Park Square, Milton Park, Abingdon, Oxon, OX14 4RN

CRC Press is an imprint of Taylor & Francis Group, LLC

Cover Artist: Lori Shields

Library of Congress Control Number: 2019948987

ISBN: 9781630917890 (hbk)
ISBN: 9781003526261 (ebk)

DOI: 10.1201/9781003526261

Dedication

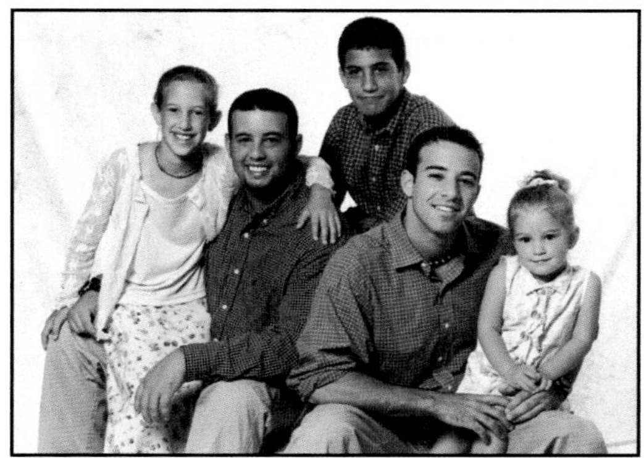

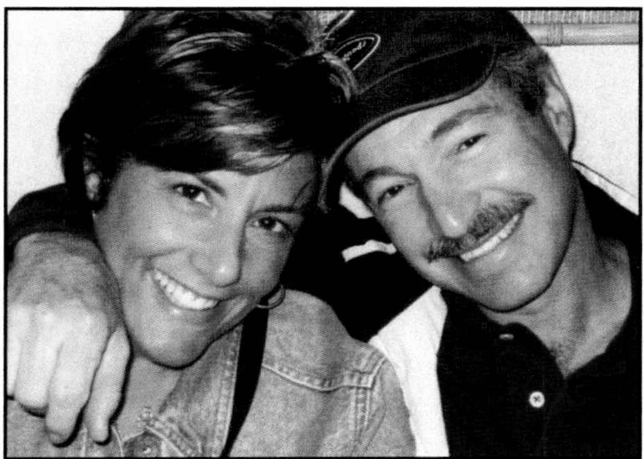

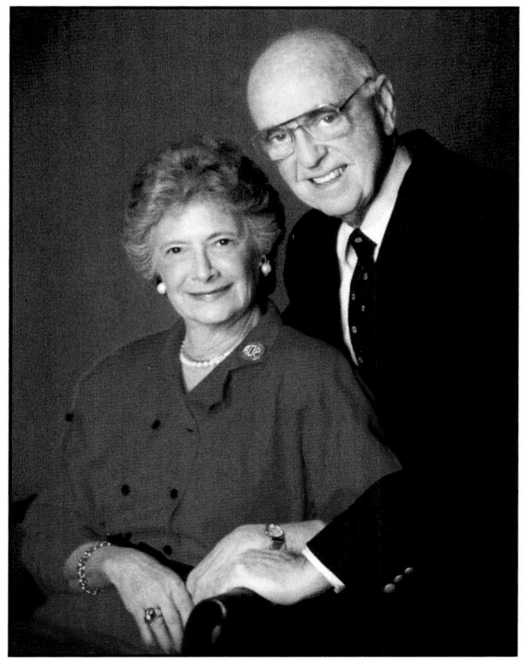

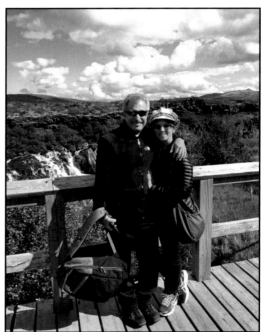

… Need I say more?

Robert H. Osher, MD

Contents

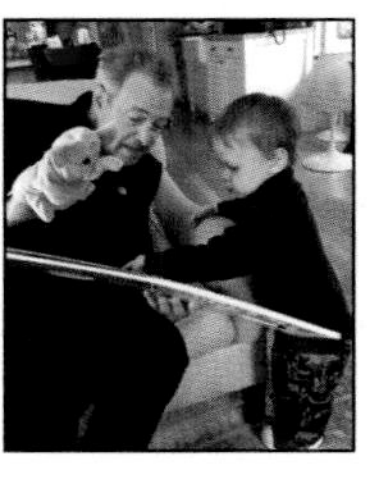

Introduction: Goals of the Real ABCs

ACHIEVEMENT

Definition of achievement: To successfully accomplish

We are all capable of significant Achievements, and this book will analyze the key ingredients that are requisite. I apologize for the flourish of trophies and awards that the reader is subjected to in the following chapters. It is not intended to reflect arrogance or braggadocio, but rather the tangible proof that the strategies for Achievement outlined by the author will pave the road to success.

BALANCE

Definition of balance: Mental or emotional equilibrium

The author admits to constant struggle in this ongoing battle. Finding Balance can be challenging for the high achiever. This book reveals a flurry of mistakes, for which I apologize to those who have been hurt by my laser focus on Achievement.

CONTENTMENT

Definition of contentment: The state, quality, or fact of being happy enough with what one has or is

Contentment is the most elusive state and the most difficult to understand. Yet, I have made considerable progress with each passing decade, and I hope to share with the reader some of the life lessons that I have learned.

Robert H. Osher, MD

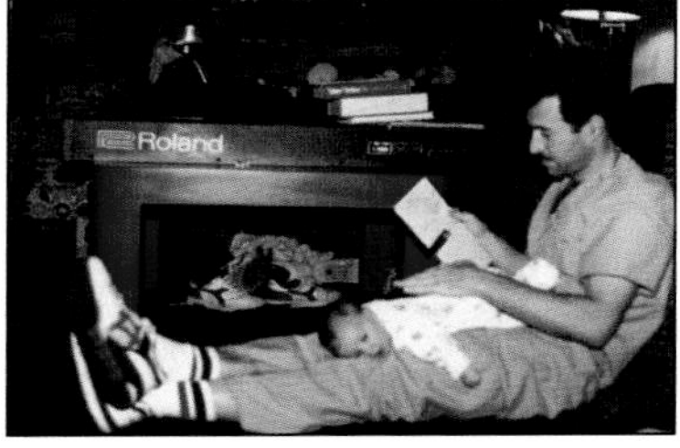

Prologue

The sound of the MRI was deafening. Even with the mandatory ear plugs, the machine gun–like sounds spinning around my head were relentless. Inside the barrel of the imaging machine, I felt like an accident victim trapped underground in a collapsed mine shaft. I was not afraid... just incredibly sad and overwhelmed by a sense of total helplessness and despair. Hours before, I had been told that I had a pineapple-sized malignant tumor in my kidney, and I was trying to cope with the death warrant I had just been issued.

There was little solace in the fact that I was a 53-year-old eye surgeon who had attained international recognition and widespread success. When facing one's own mortality, achievements mean so little, nor was I especially afraid of death, since my life had been blessed many times over. I also had a strong sense of faith, but the deepest sense of sorrow flooded my body when I thought about my 6-year-old daughter. The older children would be fine, but who would clean this little one's glasses? Who would teach her how to throw and catch? Who would be there to protect her or console her when she was teased?

The machine gun burst of the MRI abruptly ceased and was replaced by an eerie silence. My mind was racing. Fifty-three years of experiences and accumulated wisdom would likely go to waste. I had lived an extremely full life, and surely there had to be a way to pass along to my children some of the lessons that I had learned. I was about to undergo an emergency operation, and the surgeon had dutifully completed the informed consent process by acknowledging the slim chance that I would not survive this major cancer procedure. At that moment, within the MRI machine, I decided that if I survived, I would author a series of brief "lessons" to share with my loved ones, revealing the secrets on how to plan, organize, and achieve personal and professional success. Perhaps something that I would pass along would help my five children with their careers, and maybe something I wrote might also impact the quality of their lives.

I felt the sled upon which I was laying begin to move, signifying the end of the MRI. Suddenly, I felt a burst of optimism that I was going to get through this operation, and I was resolved to leave a written legacy to my children. I would tell them paragraph by paragraph what I have learned, and each child could extract what he or she considered useful toward achieving his or her own goals and developing a sense of Contentment. Let the knife fall...I have a book to write!

CHAPTER 1

Anatomy and Passion of Achievement

If there is a single characteristic shared by those who achieve, it must be the quality of passion or enthusiasm for what one is doing. Planning a strategy, initiating a task, and maintaining the momentum to get it done represent a series of significant hurdles to all, but to those armed with passion, each mandatory component in the equation for hard-earned success is easier to execute. Let's look at this equation in more detail.

First, one has to have an *imagination* before developing a *plan*. Unless one can visualize a clear starting point toward an ultimate goal, there are too many distractions and countless options that can interfere and thwart progress. Whether it is learning to play golf, creating a business model, or manufacturing a product, the components necessary to get to the end result must be visualized. Usually, daydreaming precedes the actual planning, and most everyone is capable of letting his or her mind wander from the initial idea to the finish line. In fact, for most people, it is natural to be able to visualize the reward at the end of the task. Certainly, we are each familiar with ruminations of recognition and the material gains that crown Achievement. Unfortunately, this is where most of us stop.

While dreaming of achievement is ethereal, *planning* the achievement requires concrete organization. Then, the work begins with the *initiation* of the task, another hurdle where the vast majority of us fail. We each can dream about looking fit, and we can even plan our workouts. However, initiating the task is an incredibly difficult undertaking, and failure at this point sets the stage for underachievement.

The next barrier to achievement is the issue of *perseverance*. Being disciplined and maintaining focus on the task at hand is seemingly impossible. If this were not true, everyone would be an "A" student and a high achiever. Success comes to those who understand the importance of initiating and then maintaining momentum over a prolonged period of time. Most tasks in life that lead to significant achievement cannot be completed in a single episode and require a sustained, disciplined approach. It takes years to build up muscles, acquire a degree, or rise through the hierarchy of a company. It is this requirement of invested time that is so intimidating and overwhelming. This is where passion plays such an important role.

Most of us are just not capable of going through this uphill battle without the passion necessary to fuel our focus. However, when we really love what we are doing, our passion converts an onerous task into an effortless act of pleasure. It is not only the goal at the end of the journey, but the entire journey itself that becomes enjoyable. If one has passion for planting a garden, mastering a sport, repairing a car, or learning the practice of medicine, then that individual is much more likely to succeed. This is the reason that I have always preached to my children to "find something you love to do, and then become as good as you can possibly be." Those who are lucky enough to find something that releases their passion en route to a goal are in for a successful ride on the road to Achievement.

The difficult trick is to learn how to be passionate about a seemingly unappealing task. After all, if we only did the things that we wanted to do, few people would graduate from school and even fewer would endure the labors of a post-graduate education. The ladder of success would be stunted since those at the bottom would have little interest in slowly ascending or "paying their dues" rung by rung. This is where intellectual imagination plays a wonderful role in allowing us to visualize the eventual fruits of our labor. By projecting future outcomes, it becomes easier to invest the time and effort necessary to reach nearly any goal. For example, Tiger Woods must have agonized when he underwent a major swing change despite achieving unprecedented success as an amateur. While struggling on the tour for a period of time, he was able to invest the time and effort necessary to arrive at the next level. Then, following multiple back and knee surgeries, he had to rebuild an entirely new swing. After failing over and over again, Tiger just won an epic 15th major championship. It would be fair to say that many sacrifices are made—including burning the "midnight oil" and emptying bedpans—as part of the dues that must be paid toward becoming a physician. Yet, visualizing the proverbial light at the end of the tunnel is what kept Tiger and a generation of sleep-deprived medical students trudging forward toward the goal.

Can success occur without passion? Absolutely. Being a prodigious worker is a powerful ingredient that may lead to success even when passion seems conspicuously absent. Moreover, luck is another unpredictable element (just ask the lottery winner or the guy who opened a fortune cookie that said, "Buy Apple!"). However, as a general rule, the anatomy of Achievement consists of series of concrete components including imagining or daydreaming, planning, initiating, and persevering. Hurdles and landmines abound. Success comes to those with vision, determination, discipline, and, last but not least, the passion necessary to go the distance required to achieve the goal.

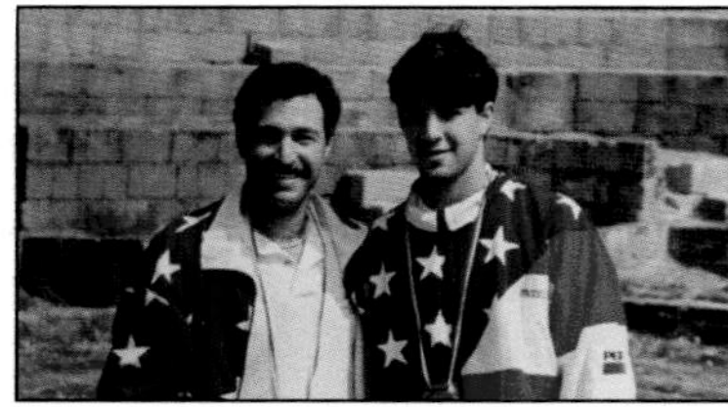

CHAPTER 2

Getting Things Accomplished

A Case Study

In 2008, while still in my 50s, I received my first Lifetime Achievement Award, this one from the American Academy of Ophthalmology (Figure 2-1). Subsequently, I was the recipient of the Kelman Award (named after the inventor or small incision cataract surgery) presented at the European Society of Cataract and Refractive Surgeons meeting in Athens, Greece (Figure 2-2). With my family by my side, I was given the Binkhorst Award, the most prestigious award from the American Society of Cataract and Refractive Surgery (Figure 2-3); the Lim Award presented at the Asia-Pacific Association of Cataract and Refractive Surgeons in China (Figure 2-4); the Gold Award, Australia's top honor (Figure 2-5); the Excellence Award from the Canadian Society of Cataract & Refractive Surgery (Figure 2-6); and the Optic Award from the Royal Society of Medicine in England (Figure 2-7). From Latin America, I received the Fundacion Oftalmologica Los Andes Award in Chile (Figure 2-8), the Kelman Award in Brazil (Figure 2-9), and an award bearing my name from the Argentinean Society of Cataract and Refractive Surgery (Figure 2-10). I am the proud recipient of 40 awards in the international cataract video competitions (Figure 2-11). The most recent award is a Lifetime Achievement Award from the American Osteopathic Colleges of Ophthalmology and Otolaryngology Head & Neck Surgery (Figure 2-12). There have been many other awards and moments of recognition along the way.

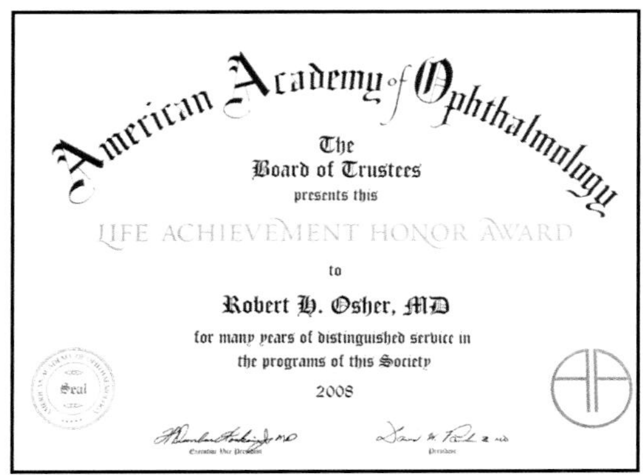
American Academy of Ophthalmology
The Board of Trustees
presents this
LIFE ACHIEVEMENT HONOR AWARD
to
Robert H. Osher, MD
for many years of distinguished service in
the programs of this Society
2008
Seal

Figure 2-1. Lifetime Achievement Award from the American Academy of Ophthalmology.

While I can clearly define the specific ingredients for Achievement that have helped me, only you can "roll up your sleeves" and get the job done in your own unique manner. My professional career and personal lifestyle may not be "right" for anyone else. Nevertheless, you may be able to use my life as a case study when it comes to how to get things accomplished.

I finished my ophthalmic training at the Bascom Palmer Eye Institute in Miami, Florida and the Wills Eye Hospital in Philadelphia, Pennsylvania, the top two programs in ophthalmology ranked by the *U.S. News & World Report*, and I had decided to complete several elective fellowships that would provide additional expertise in my chosen field. I worked very hard and published a variety of scientific articles, which gave me a strong head start in the race up the career

Osher RH. *The Real ABCs: A Surgeon's Analysis and a Father's Legacy, Second Edition* (pp 3-17).

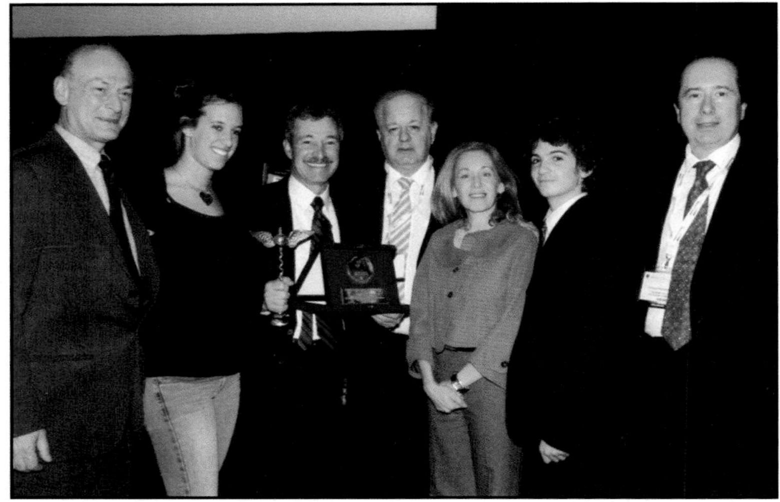

Figure 2-2. Kelman Award from the Hellenic Society with my daughter, Jenny, and Ann Kelman, wife of the late Dr. Charles Kelman.

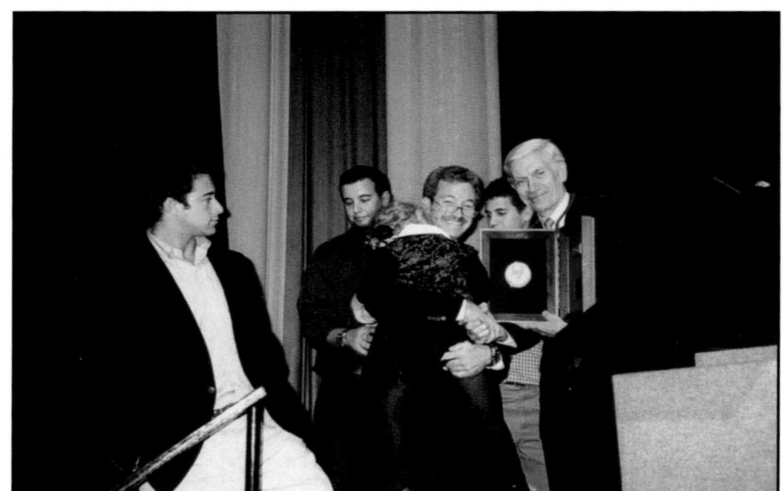

Figure 2-3. Binkhorst Award from the American Society of Cataract and Refractive Surgery with a bigger award, daughter, Jessie, asleep on my shoulder, along with my three sons, Jeff, James, and Jon.

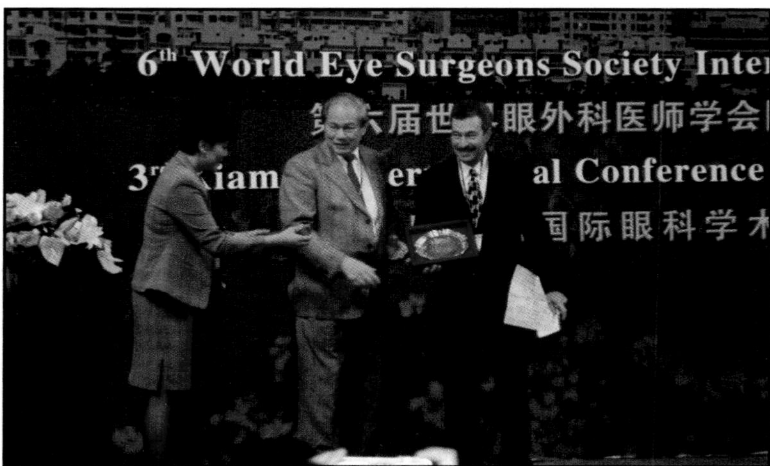

Figure 2-4. Lim Award from the Asia-Pacific Association of Cataract and Refractive Surgeons, presented by the late Dr. Arthur Lim.

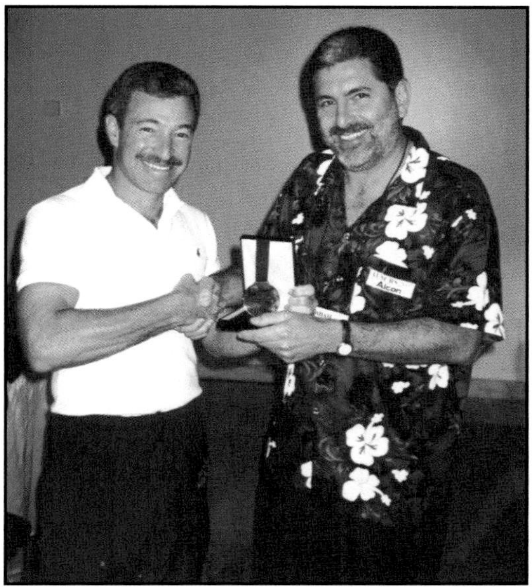

Figure 2-5. Gold Award from the Australia Society of Cataract and Refractive Surgeons presented by President Graham Barrett, MD.

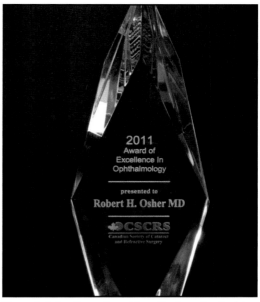

Figure 2-6. Excellence Award from the Canadian Society of Cataract & Refractive Surgery.

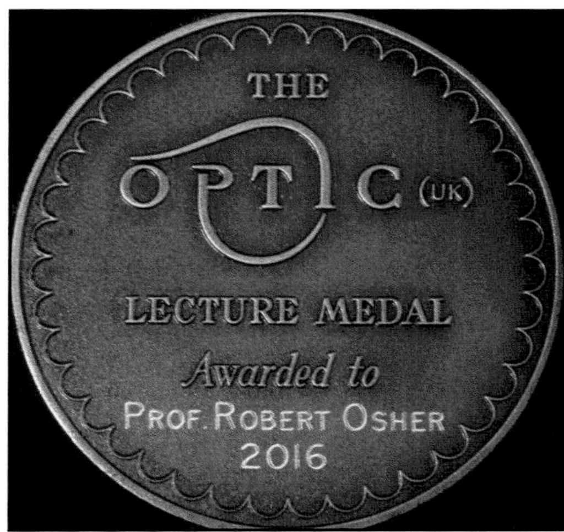

Figure 2-7. Optic Award from the Royal Society of Medicine in England.

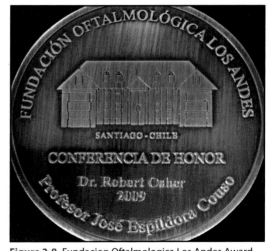

Figure 2-8. Fundacion Oftalmologica Los Andes Award from Chile.

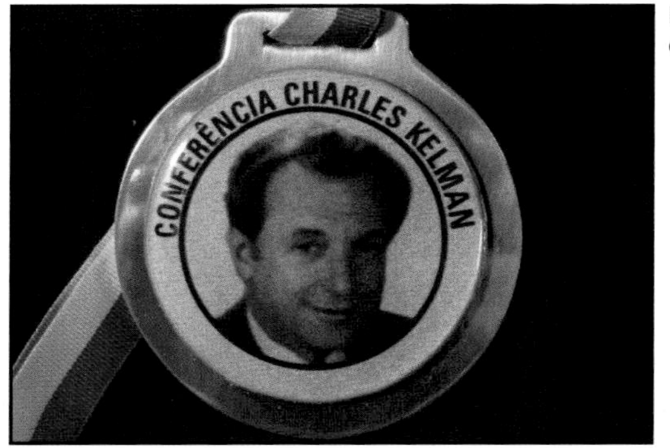

Figure 2-9. Kelman Award from the Brazilian Society of Cataract and Refractive Surgery.

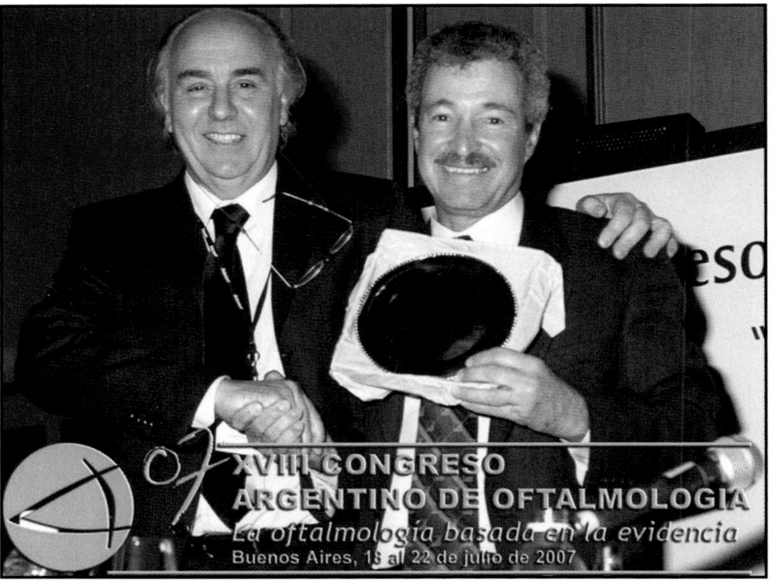

Figure 2-10. Inaugural Osher Lectureship in Argentina, presented by the late president, Dr. Carlos Argento.

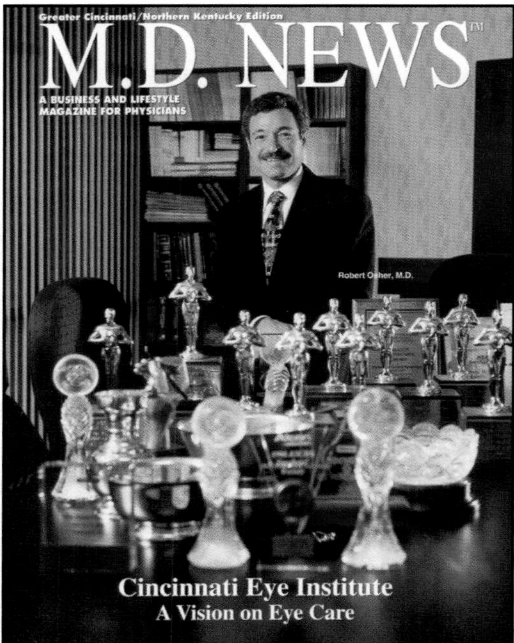

Figure 2-11. Cover of MD News circa 2000.

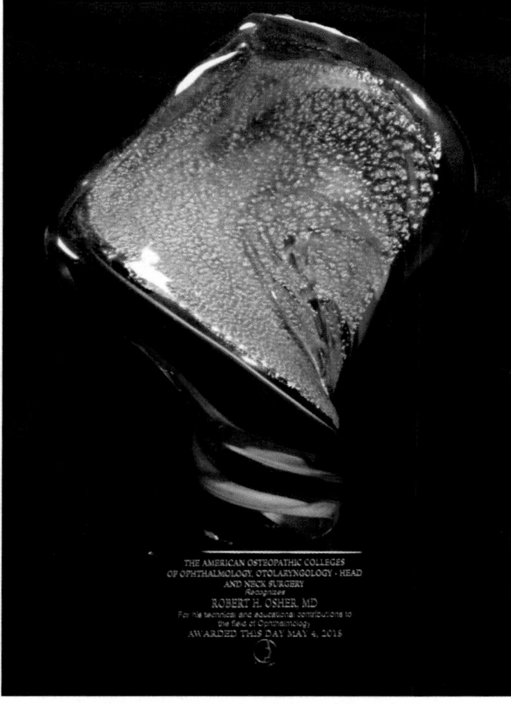

Figure 2-12. American Osteopathic Colleges of Ophthalmology and Otolaryngology Head & Neck Surgery Award.

ladder. I was well prepared to select a teaching position at a prestigious university and begin an ascent that would eventually take me to the top of the academic ivory tower. However, I had a recurrent fear that once at the top, I would look around and realize that I had spent a career climbing the wrong ladder! While the ego gratification of making an unusual diagnosis in front

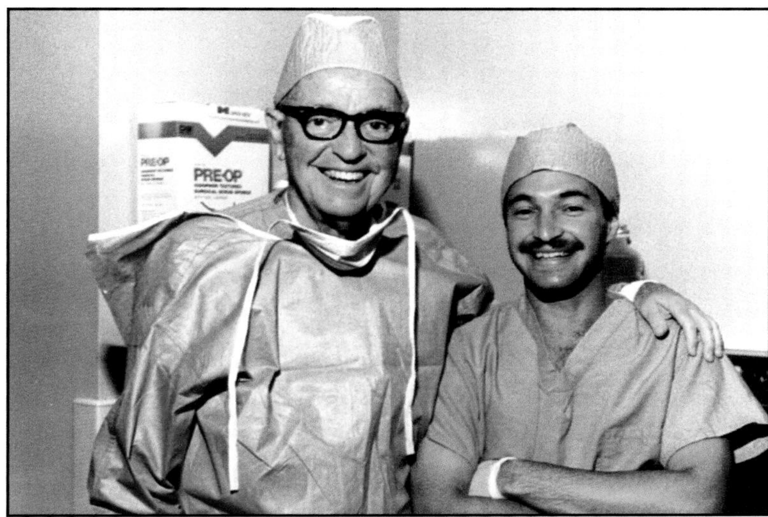

Figure 2-13. Morris S. Osher, MD —my hero—invited me to come home after three fellowships and spend 6 months with Dad. We practiced together for 18 years.

of a group of medical students was satisfying, it seemed more rewarding for me to participate in everyday patient care. In other words, I realized that I would rather deal with patients than be a full-time professor.

Morris Osher, MD, my father and a very special physician, proposed that I return to Cincinnati, Ohio to spend 6 months working in his office and delay my career decision for a while longer (Figure 2-13). After 12 years away, I returned to Cincinnati eager to determine where my career was headed, and it did not take much time to find out. After accompanying my father to the operating room and watching him perform exquisite cataract surgery and then observing the ecstatic patient when the patch came off, I had discovered what I wanted to do for the rest of my life.

Cataract surgery is incredible! We are born with a crystal-clear lens that is about the size of an M&M,* which is suspended inside the eye by tiny spider web–like structures. From moment to moment throughout our lives, the lens changes shape to precisely focus incoming light onto the retina much like the way the lens in a camera focuses the image onto the film. As we age (and rarely from other causes), this transparent lens begins to cloud or opacify, which is the definition of a cataract (Figure 2-14).

As the cataract advances, the patient notices a decrease in vision along with glare and halos. When the visual symptoms are no longer acceptable, the patient can elect to undergo cataract surgery. Either under a local anesthetic or using just a few drops to numb the eye, the cataract is removed through an incision only 2 mm in length, smaller than the width of a pencil (Figure 2-15). This is accomplished by breaking the cataract into tiny pieces with ultrasonic energy and then vacuuming these fragments out of the eye. Next, the cloudy cataractous lens is replaced with a crystal clear artificial lens that not only focuses, but also contains a built-in sunglass. Because it can be scrolled up like a newspaper, it is inserted through the same tiny incision and placed into position, where it remains invisible behind the iris, the colored part of the eye (Figure 2-16). The incision is so small that stitches are not required. This elegant operation is painless and bloodless, and I have enjoyed showing the live surgery to the accompanying family on a closed-circuit monitor for almost 4 decades. The patient no longer needs hospitalization nor even an eye patch, and, by the next day, his or her vision is usually good enough to pass a driver's test without glasses.

* Mars, Inc

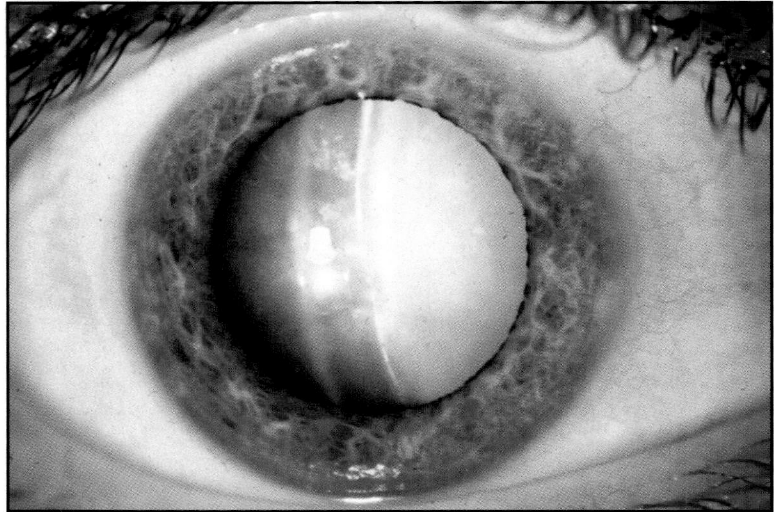

Figure 2-14. A cataract is a loss of transparency of the human lens.

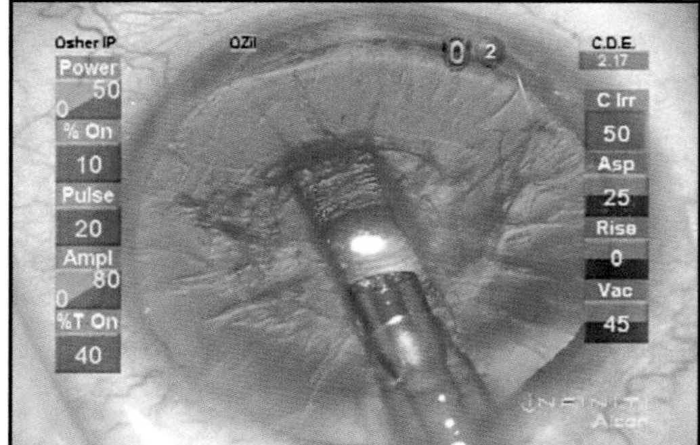

Figure 2-15. Phacoemulsification is the microincisional ultrasonic removal of a cataract.

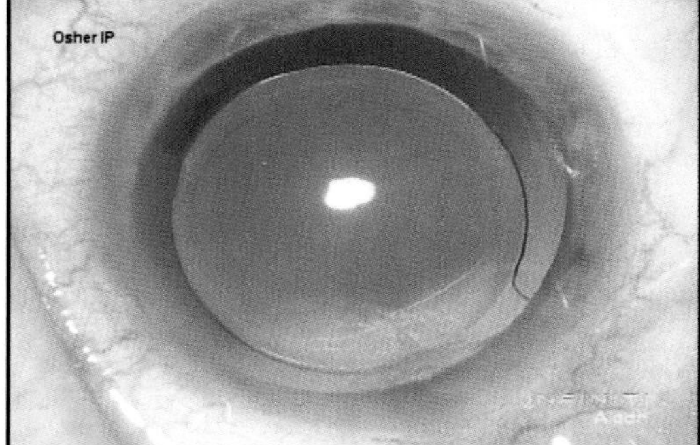

Figure 2-16. Intraocular lens implanted to restore vision.

What in the entire universe could possibly be more gratifying than helping a nearly blind patient recover clear vision on the day following surgery? It is astonishing for the patient and extremely satisfying for the surgeon.

So, I found my niche. My father helped me get started by referring quite a few of his patients who needed cataract surgery. As my experience and confidence grew, I wanted to devote my life to just 4 mm of tissue! I was no longer interested in being a general ophthalmologist like everyone else, a jack of all trades, and master of none. The big question was how could I limit my entire practice to this wonderful operation? Then, the idea hit me with the subtlety of an avalanche. Why not develop an institute composed of physicians who would dedicate their entire careers to each of the ophthalmic subspecialties? Would it be possible to build a private practice by recruiting a team of pure experts in glaucoma, retina, cornea, pediatric ophthalmology, inflammation, oculoplastics, ophthalmic oncology, refractive surgery, neuro-ophthalmology, medical eye care, and even emergency ophthalmology?

The more I thought about it, the more interesting this concept became. A subspecialty practice was not uncommon in a university setting, but it was unheard of in private practice. Moreover, in the early 1980s, there were no practices limited to cataract surgery. I realized that we needed a building to get started. This building would require special construction that would allow each subspecialist to design his or her own area in a manner that would permit optimal patient care and efficient patient flow through the maze of waiting rooms, exam lanes, and special testing. Moreover, our own ambulatory surgery center would need to be housed inside of this building because a hospital could not possibly accommodate ophthalmic subspecialty surgical requirements in the same facility that caters to appendectomies and hysterectomies. I was confident that an operating theater could be designed that would provide the ideal combination of "high tech" and "high touch" for each subspecialist. I envisioned families of patients being able to participate by viewing the actual surgical procedures, another radical idea.

Before any of these dreams could be possible, I had to approach my father and his three partners in order to convince them that a major paradigm shift in direction would be in everyone's best interest. My father suggested that we create a new position that would be called "Medical Director," probably in an attempt to appease me. Perhaps he thought that a fancy title would suppress my desire to explore unchartered waters, but I continued to badger the group into giving my idea a try. That's when another senior partner suggested that we retain a consulting group with expertise in performing psychological testing on executives. After submitting to 3 days of intensive evaluations, I can vividly recall the evening when the physicians gathered around our oval mahogany table, listening intently to the test results. It was explained that I was quite average in most aptitudes, but measured off the bell-shaped curve in two specific areas. My associates were informed that my AMBITION titer was off the scale, which made beads of sweat appear on their foreheads. However, a collective sigh of relief followed when they were informed that I had achieved the highest marks ever recorded in the category of LOYALTY. It must have been quite reassuring to know that the new Medical Director was crazed with ambition but was as loyal as a puppy! This landmark meeting ended with a somewhat reluctant vote of confidence, and I was officially given the green light to move forward with my ideas for building the first private eye institute in our part of the country.

Now, I could roll up my sleeves and get to work. The plan conceived in 1980 was set in motion, and I began recruiting pure ophthalmic subspecialists, real experts in their respective fields. I described my vision to each applicant and enthusiastically concluded the interview with a simple philosophy pertaining to our future institute: "If we build it, they will come," paraphrasing the theme of the movie *Field of Dreams*. I meticulously researched each applicant's track record, calling every co-resident in their ophthalmology training program. I reasoned that an "apple-polisher" or a "brown-noser" could easily fool the faculty, but those who knew the applicant best were his or her co-workers from down in the trenches. I also called the nursing staff that had worked with the applicant, who could bring a unique perspective about the applicant's "true colors." Long-winded curriculum vitaes were ignored since I was only interested in the answers to four basic questions. First, was the applicant highly qualified and highly skilled? Second, was the applicant completely honest and a person of integrity? Third, was the applicant a prodigious worker who would not shy away from hard work? Fourth, would this "star" be a prima donna or a team player? This research paid off big dividends, and I began hiring an enormously talented and highly compatible group of subspecialists.

In the meantime, a simultaneous project was launched to identify an ideal location to build the home of the future Cincinnati Eye Institute. I had selected this name to serve as an umbrella for patient care, an educational center, a research facility, and an ambulatory surgery center. Somehow, we had to stay connected to the rest of the medical world without isolating ourselves in some commercial outlet mall. Lady Luck was on my side when I met Thomas Wilburn, President of the Bethesda Hospitals in Cincinnati. Mr. Wilburn had already established his reputation as a health care visionary when he positioned the Bethesda System as the most successful model in our region. He listened carefully as I described my concept of a full-service subspecialty eye institute that could add another jewel to his impressive crown of accomplishments in exchange for what I perceived to be the finest location in Cincinnati.

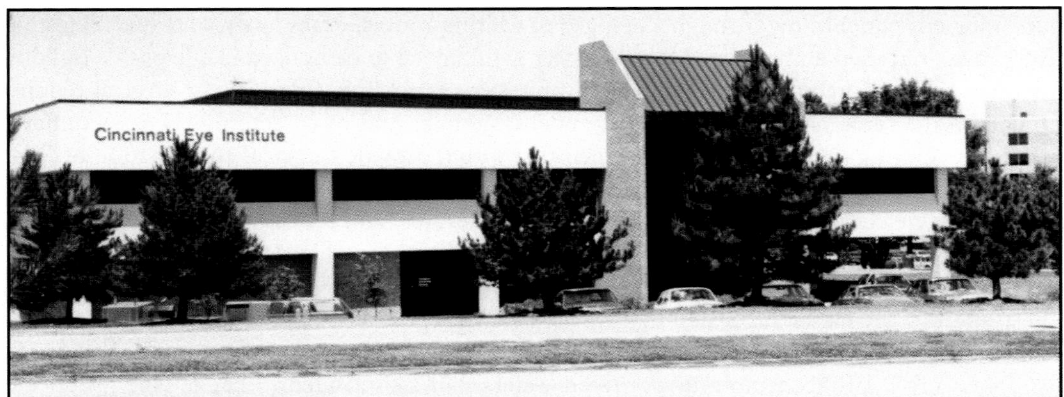

Figure 2-17. CEI circa 1984.

Not only did Mr. Wilburn shake my hand with sincerity and enthusiasm, but he offered the very best site in front of his very best hospital. Rarely have I shaken the hand of a man to whom I felt so grateful. I could visualize the institute even before a single blade of grass was displaced.

The next hurdle was gaining regulatory approval for the ambulatory surgery center. This was a politically charged issue because the competing hospitals were so powerful that they could veto the granting of a Certificate of Need by simply claiming that an additional freestanding ambulatory surgical center was unnecessary. Despite approaching high-level health care officials, congressmen, and wealthy benefactors, I could not find a single ally outside of Mr. Wilburn. The responses varied from "Who needs it!" to "Are you trying to hurt the hospital?" Fortunately, there was an attorney, Bob Brant, who was as obsessive-compulsive as me, and he was able to find a loophole in the state regulations. If we did not administer "general anesthesia" nor designate a "dedicated recovery room," we could circumvent the state requirements for a Certificate of Need. This was wonderful news since ophthalmic surgery does not require general anesthesia. Moreover, I always had detested the concept of a dedicated recovery room. I wanted my patients to have their own pre- and postoperative area to share with their loved ones, privately and with dignity. All of the pieces were beginning to fall into place.

Physicians usually make poor administrators, and I was no exception. Again, Lady Luck was at my side when a young accountant named Doris Holton demonstrated reliability, integrity, and an extraordinary work ethic. My father was usually an excellent judge of character, and he recommended that I select Doris as my administrative partner. She would be able to get things accomplished while I was taking care of patients. Achievement is often easier when there is a team approach, especially when the leader trusts those around him or her to get the job done. The risk of this "blind" trust is being deceived or embezzled, which actually happened years later when I hired David, a real con man, to work with Doris.

To make a long story short and to condense 2 decades into several paragraphs, we had arrived at a winning formula. A 50,000-square foot building served as the new home of the Cincinnati Eye Institute (CEI; Figure 2-17). The recruited physicians and surgeons were outstanding, and each became very successful while contributing to the growing reputation of our referral eye center. Then, the dean of the local medical school requested help with his stagnant ophthalmology department, which led to my integrating his group of talented subspecialists into our roster. Our staff grew from the original handful to nearly 50 ophthalmologists and 500 employees, with multiple offices in three states. Within several years, CEI had become the largest private practice ophthalmology group in the United States. Eventually, we outgrew our building and had to find another home: this time 114,767 square feet, including seven operating rooms (Figure 2-18).

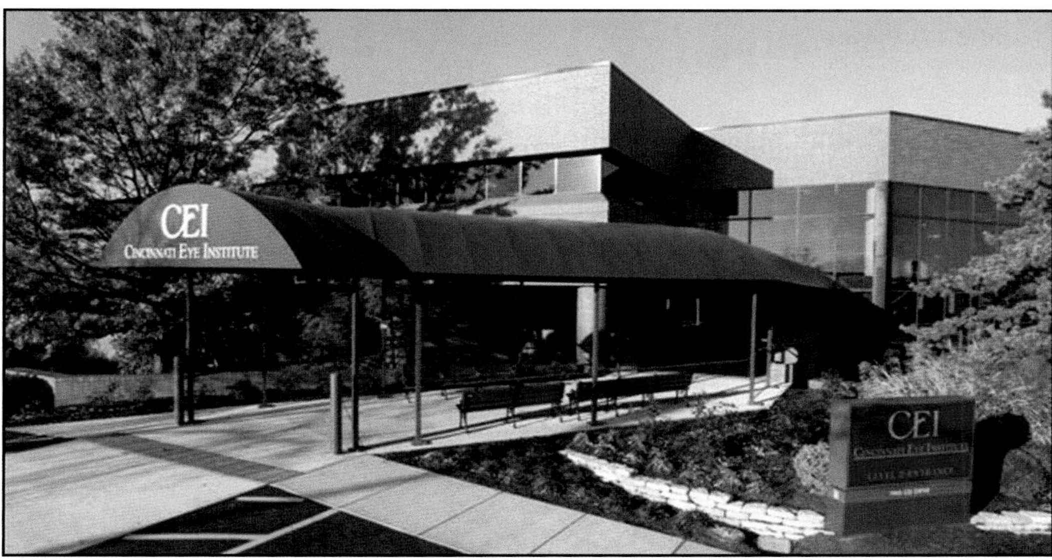

Figure 2-18. CEI 2019.

FROM YOUR MEDICAL DIRECTOR . . .

The Cincinnati Eye Institute will be the leader in Ophthalmology by providing the highest quality ophthalmic care and related services. We will conduct our practice according to the highest ethical standards keeping foremost in our thoughts that patient satisfaction is our most important objective. Our daily decisions and activities must continually serve this goal.

Robert H. Osher, M.D.

Figure 2-19. Our mission was crystal clear! This sign was located just inside the employee entrance.

From the beginning, CEI raised the bar for excellence in high-tech, compassionate patient care. Our first surgery center contained four state-of-the-art operating rooms with top-of-the-line equipment and instrumentation, much of which we designed. A broadcast-quality video system allowed us to televise and record each surgery for teaching purposes, while allowing us to narrate the operation for the accompanying family members. At the conclusion of the operation, the family would be awaiting the patient's return to their private recovery room in which embraces and lots of love were exchanged.

The clinical facilities were also designed for patient comfort. The subspecialty waiting rooms permitted patients with similar conditions to mingle. Postoperative patients reassured those who were waiting for preoperative consultations. Spacious skylights, large screen televisions playing patient educational material, coffee and snacks, and, of course, a rose for each surgical patient were just some of the amenities for which we received glowing evaluations in our patient surveys. There is an old expression that was proving to be true: "Patients do not care how much you know until they know how much you care!" I posted this reminder and others on the wall of the employee entrance and in each employee restroom during my 20-year tenure as Medical Director (Figure 2-19).

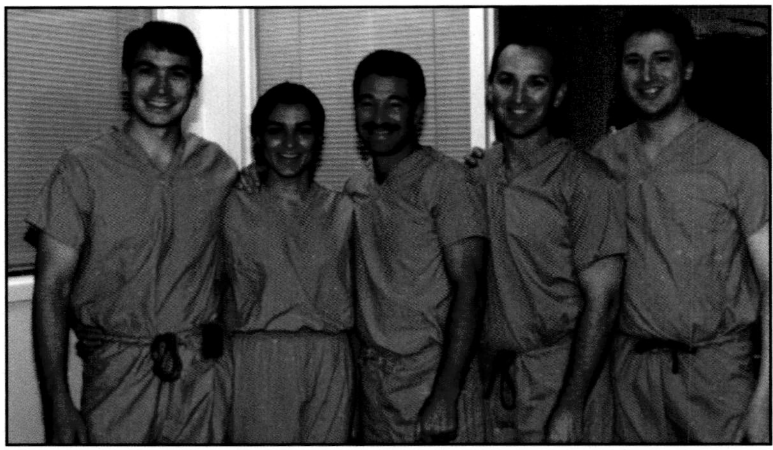

Figure 2-20. CEI Cataract Team: Drs. Burk, DaMata, Osher, Cionni, and Snyder. Missing: Dr. James Faulkner.

Even though CEI had become a model for many medical practices around the country, I never derived nearly as much satisfaction from the work invested in building our organization as I enjoyed from patient care. I always took great pride in taking a careful history, performing a thorough examination, and offering the patient an unrushed explanation. Since all of my patients were referred by other ophthalmologists and optometrists, I dictated a comprehensive report to the referring doctor at the conclusion of the examination and then answered any final questions from the patient or the family. I scheduled only one or two new patients each hour since my patients were often extremely complex and coming from different cities, states, and countries. If a patient needed more time, I gave it willingly. I had the same thorough approach in the operating room and refused to yield to the pressure of scheduling more and more patients, working faster and faster. I viewed each operation as a work of art, for which I would prepare diligently the evening before. Visiting surgeons were impressed that every step of every procedure had to be just right. Meticulous surgical technique with excellent results in combination with loving care delivered by a devoted and compassionate staff caused my practice to explode. After several years, I was performing over 1000 operations each year. I was thrilled to share my growing surgical volume with a few talented young surgeons, Dr. Bob Cionni, Dr. Mike Snyder, and Dr. Scott Burk, who I had either trained or recruited to join the cataract team (Figure 2-20). Drs. Cionni and Snyder eventually became renowned surgeons, receiving the highest awards in our specialty. We lost Dr. Burk to a brain glioblastoma, but not before this brilliant young surgeon had introduced several techniques that changed our approach to managing surgical complications by visualizing invisible structures like the vitreous gel and epiretinal membranes. His loss was devastating to me.

While my role as a surgeon and CEI Medical Director often seemed like two full-time jobs, I made another major commitment early in my career. After finishing my fellowship training, I decided to devote one-third of my time to teaching, a wonderful way to give back to the profession. My definition of teaching was broad as it included lecturing, publishing, and producing educational videos. However, in order to lecture, it is necessary to be invited to lecture, so I had to begin building a reputation. In 1980, every eye surgeon who spoke at the podium would only show his most beautiful cases. I took the opposite approach and established the first Video Symposium, a forum in which only difficult patients and complications were demonstrated. I reasoned that every surgeon, no matter how talented, would occasionally encounter a challenging situation or an unanticipated complication. Because I let the video recorder run during the entirety of every operation, it was astonishing how many unique situations were captured

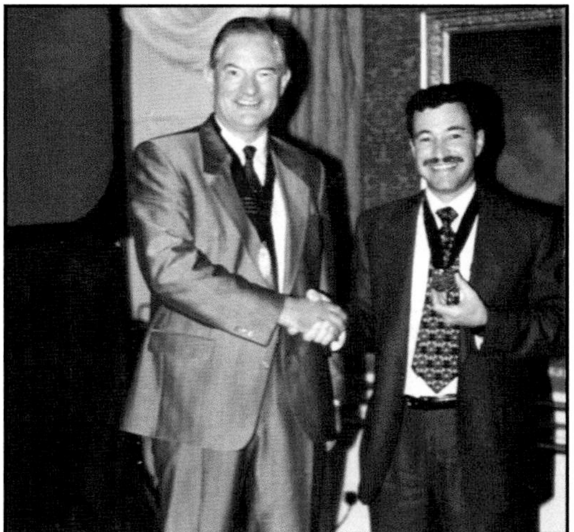

Figure 2-21. Rayner Medal from the United Kingdom Intraocular Implant Society.

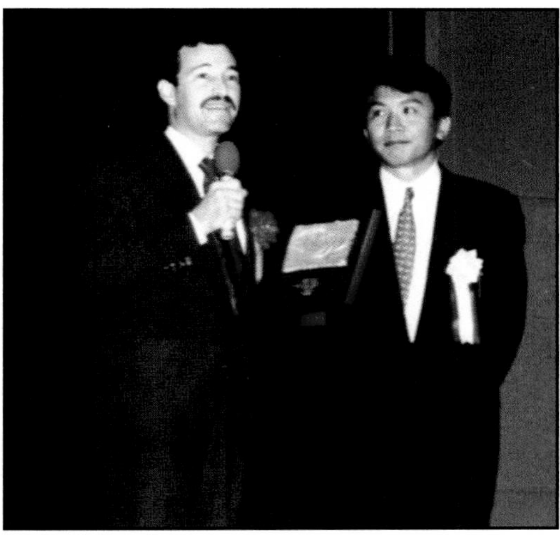

Figure 2-22. Canon Award in Japan.

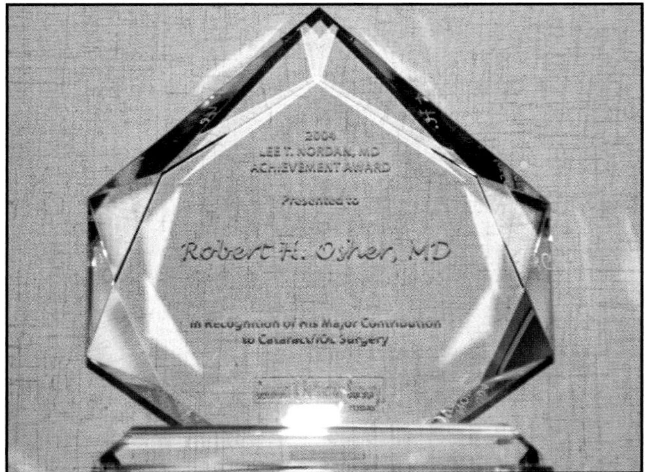

Figure 2-23. Nordan Award from *Cataract & Refractive Surgery Today*.

on tape. I had enough self-confidence that I did not mind showing my complications since each was managed to the best of my ability. Moreover, I knew that the educational benefit to the audience was unsurpassed. My courses rapidly grew in attendance and became among the largest offered at the major American, European, and Latin American meetings. My personal lecture itinerary expanded to a grueling 100,000 miles/year of travel, which included honorary lectureships in more than 40 countries. In addition to some of the awards mentioned previously, I was the recipient of the Rayner Medal from England (Figure 2-21), the Canon Award from Japan (Figure 2-22), the Nordan Award (Figure 2-23) and the Maumenee Award (Figure 2-24) in America, the Mooney Award from Ireland (Figure 2-25), and the coveted Innovator's Award from the American Society of Cataract and Refractive Surgery (Figure 2-26). It really did not matter to me whether there were 10 surgeons or 1000 surgeons in the audience. If someone could benefit from my surgical experience, the trip was worthwhile. I can vividly recall traveling to places like Buenos Aires, Argentina; Tokyo, Japan; and Auckland, New Zealand just to give several hours of presentations and then, immediately upon finishing my lectures, I was in a taxi heading back to the airport to fly home!

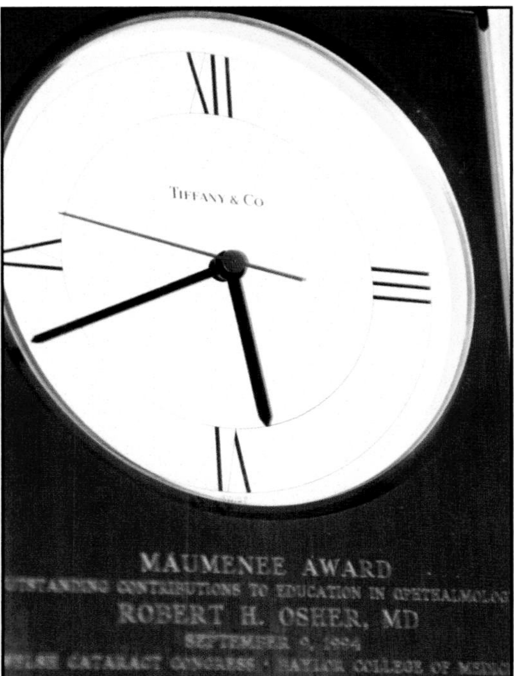

Figure 2-24. Maumenee Award from the Cataract Congress.

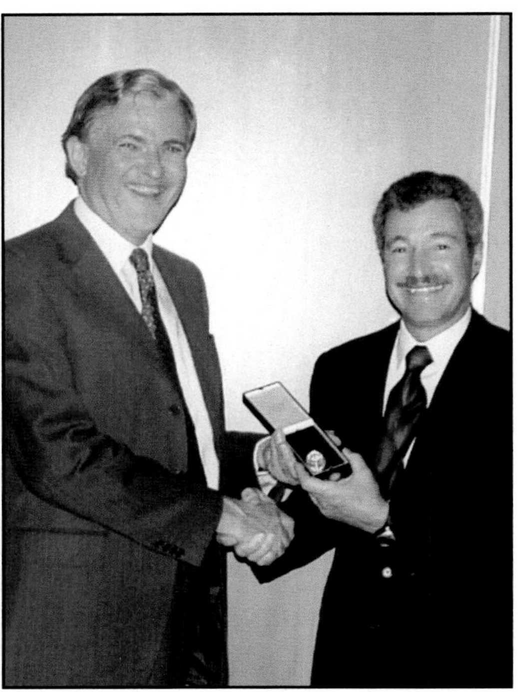

Figure 2-25. Mooney Award from the Irish College of Ophthalmologists.

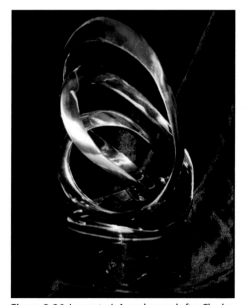

Figure 2-26. Innovator's Award named after Charles Kelman, MD, inventor of phacoemulsification.

Scientific publications represent the backbone of medical progress and individual contribution. Yet, writing a journal article, chapter, or book requires an unbelievable amount of time. I developed a successful strategy in order to be able to publish. First, I kept detailed files and videos of all interesting and unusual cases, even when I was unsure of the diagnosis or surgical management. Second, I set a goal to write an article that would be submitted for publication every 4 to 6 months, in some years publishing as many as 12 peer-reviewed articles. Third, I would take the preliminary draft of the article with me and invest some quality time during every plane ride. Fourth, I would invite a Fellow or partner to collaborate, easing the burden of collecting references, making illustrations, or taking photographs. Finally, I would work on the article by dictating a paragraph when driving in my car to pick up a child or when going to a countless number of sporting events. By utilizing this significant amount of time that would otherwise be wasted on mindless radio, a steady stream of publications was always flowing into the ophthalmic literature. I even managed to co-author or contribute to 40 books on cataract surgery by dictating on treadmills, on exercycles, and during halftimes!

Perhaps the most significant educational project I have been involved in was the founding of the *Video Journal of Cataract and Refractive Surgery* in the early 1980s (Figure 2-27). This journal

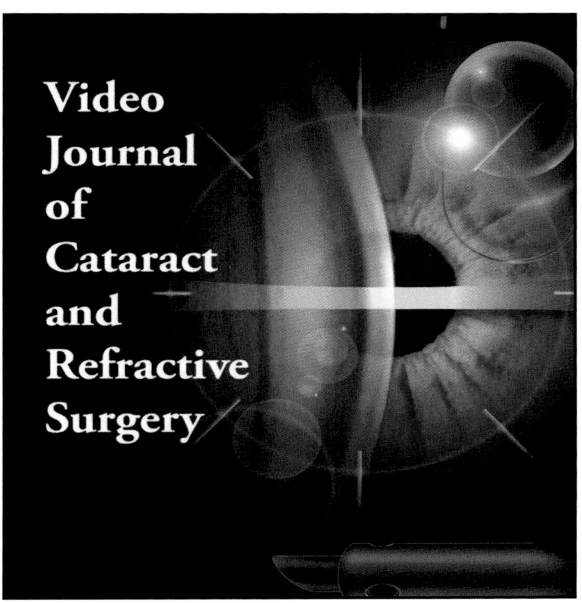

Figure 2-27. *Video Journal of Cataract and Refractive Surgery*, which I founded and have served as Editor for more than 35 years.

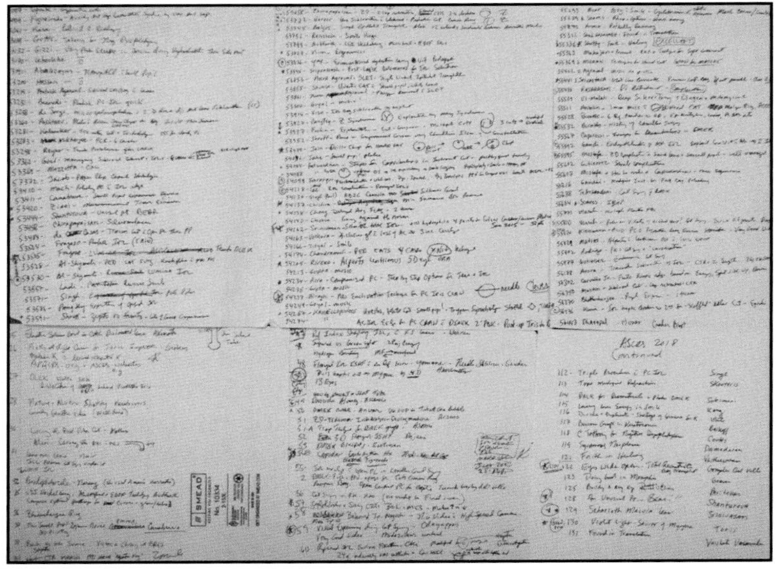

Figure 2-28. Taking notes on hundreds of videos every year.

was the first video journal in medicine with hour-long, quarterly programs featuring a variety of surgical techniques and innovations from the leading surgeons around the planet. The viewing surgeon would benefit because he or she would be able to learn new surgical procedures in the comfort of home without incurring traveling expenses or lost time away from the office. This learning approach predated the internet by decades. Moreover, the editor (me) would benefit by seeing everything, as I would watch 300 to 400 surgical videos each year (Figure 2-28). This allowed me to stay on the "cutting edge," and enjoy the enormous satisfaction of helping surgeons incorporate the best possible techniques for their patients. The *Video Journal* eventually became a free member benefit of the cataract societies in Europe (ESCRS), Asia (APAO and AUSPRS), Australia, Canada (COS), and Latin America (PAAO), attracting an international viewership of 30,000 surgeons. So much work, but so worth it!

Scientific and clinical research has also been very important to me. For almost 4 decades, I have enjoyed investigating new devices, intraocular lenses, medications, instruments, and machines for cataract surgery. Working with animal or cadaver eyes in the laboratory or assessing the performance of a new lens implant in surgery has kept me on my toes and reinforced my desire to contribute to my chosen specialty. Frankly, it has been exciting and satisfying to be able to influence the direction of eye surgery. Fortune 500 companies identified my enthusiasm and strong work ethic, which resulted in a number of consulting opportunities for prestigious companies such as Pfizer, Novartis, 3M, Johnson & Johnson, Allergan, Bausch + Lomb, Pharmacia, Abbott Medical Optics, Zeiss, Becton Dickinson, and Alcon. Later in my career, I decided to decline many relationships with industry because I was invited to chair multiple symposia on new products, and I did not want to be vulnerable to having a conflict of interest. Yet, my experience has shown that progress is more likely to occur when surgeons work closely with industry toward a shared goal.

Another small but fascinating part of my early medical practice was serving as an expert witness in malpractice trials. Several times each year, I would receive a stack of medical records from an attorney or an insurance company requesting that I render an opinion. Regardless of whether I was retained by the patient or by the physician, it was very interesting to comb through the records in painstaking detail, attempting to reconstruct the events that led to the litigation. While I tried to be brutally honest in my interpretation of the records, I soon realized that in the field of malpractice law, right and wrong are often camouflaged by the smoke and mirrors of a smooth-talking attorney. Eventually, I grew frustrated with the unfairness of the legal system and I stopped reviewing cases, but I would often count my blessings that I was able to practice medicine rather than law for a living. Caring for patients is so interesting and satisfying that, were it not for the sinister insurance industry and unscrupulous malpractice attorneys, I am convinced that nearly everyone would seek a career in medicine.

After 20 years of serving as the Medical Director, I stepped aside to concentrate on my own cataract practice. Honestly, I was very happy to turn over my role to a newly-formed Board of Directors, consisting of nine elected surgeons. One more meeting with a hospital or insurance company might have killed me! CEI continued to grow under new and more talented leadership with a new building, multiple surgery centers, and more than 600 employees. The high point was when my second son, Jamey, joined the practice as our 10th retinal surgeon. A prodigious worker, superb diagnostician, and skillful surgeon, I have enjoyed watching his referral practice grow like wildfire. I attend his conferences with the residents who appreciate his strong commitment to their education. Recently, Jamey was elected to the CEI Board of Directors and became President of the Cincinnati Society of Ophthalmology; the torch has been passed (Figure 2-29). The low point, I fear, was when the group decided to partner with private equity, a decision that I hope will allow our surgeons to continue delivering the highest-quality of care, maintaining the camaraderie of the group, and remaining capable of attracting the most talented, young ophthalmologists. We have never worked with big business, and I am concerned that our goals may not be aligned. Time will tell.

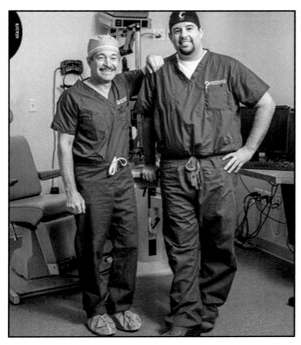

Figure 2-29. Third-generation ophthalmologist, my son Jamey.

I am now the oldest surgeon at CEI, and I admit that I am an anachronism. I still love caring for my patients and performing cataract surgery in my slow but meticulous way, and I continue to give each new patient 45 minutes of time and my cell phone number. I am not very productive in terms of generating revenue, but I am very happy. One should never confuse net worth and self-worth. My partners periodically ask about my plans for retirement, and I reply that I have an exit strategy: death! Even though I am in the final stages of my career, I believe that I am the luckiest old guy in the universe, and I count my blessings to be able to do what I do every day. However, this book is not about luck; it is about exploring and understanding the pathways that are likely to lead to Achievement and success. Let's try to dissect some of the components that are conducive to reaching one's goals.

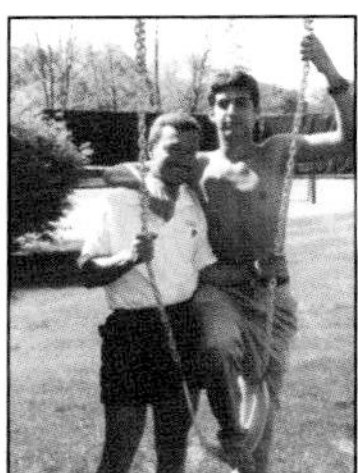

CHAPTER 3

Prepare to Succeed

Success rarely comes by accident. Yet, it is astonishing that such a simple truism has eluded so many: success is achieved by rigorous preparation. I am amused by the ongoing philosophical debate that centers around the question of whether genetic or environmental factors are more contributory to an individual's success. As far as I am concerned, the debate should be banned since the answer is so obvious. Success is a matter of hard work, and then, more hard work.

I understand that each of us is born with certain attributes and limitations. For example, I stand 5'6" (on my toes), and it would not be reasonable for me to define success as playing basketball in the NBA. However, I made the high school basketball team, played fraternity ball in college, and then led my medical school team to the hospital championship as a result of hard work alone. I clearly recall that my high school coach was quick to point out that I had neither quickness nor height—assets that cannot be taught. Yet, I could shoot the lights out because I loved to practice. During medical school, every evening I would leave the library at about 11:00 pm, hustle down to the gym, which was in the basement of Strong Memorial Hospital, and then shoot for 1 solid hour. I believe that I reached my personal basketball potential, which satisfied my individual and reasonable definition of success on the court.

That is not to say that remarkable accomplishments cannot be achieved by extraordinary efforts in sports or in any other walk of life. I had the pleasure of coaching a youngster named Kevin Youkilis for 6 or 7 years. He was an above-average athlete who was not a gifted physical specimen. Yet, he loved baseball more than any kid on the planet, and he worked relentlessly at improving his fundamentals. One year, we qualified to represent the State of Ohio in the National Championships in Tarkio, Missouri. The top baseball players from across the country were present, and Kevin did not stand out by any means, except for his intense desire and unrivaled work ethic. He practiced constantly with his devoted father, Mike, who was never too tired to throw Kevin hours and hours of batting practice. Kevin went on to set many of the records at the University of Cincinnati. After joining the Boston Red Sox, he was voted onto the American League All Star roster three times and won a Gold Glove for his defense, the Hank Aaron Award for his slugging, and a World Series ring. Kevin was recently inducted into the Red Sox Hall of Fame; not bad for a kid who was cut from the junior high school team (Figure 3-1)!

The basic principle is just undeniable. If one works hard enough, then success is almost inevitable. The basketball teams that I coached were rarely the most talented, but we were extremely successful, achieving seven consecutive AAU Ohio State Championships, reaching the Final Four twice at the National Championships (Figure 3-2) because we were always so well prepared. We might have reviewed the same in-bound play dozens of times in a practice until it was

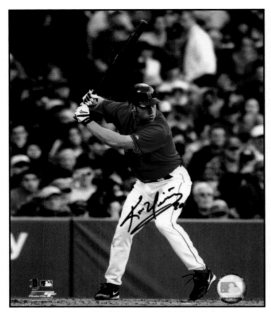

Figure 3-1. Boston Red Sox star Kevin Youkilis' success was the result of his incredible work ethic.

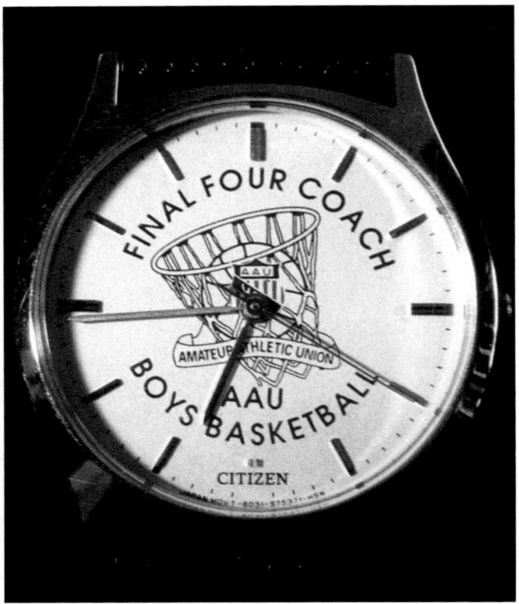

Figure 3-2. Memorabilia from reaching the Final Four twice at the National Championships.

run with exact precision. I knew that perfect practice leads to predictable execution on the court when it counts. The same applies to the operating room, where practicing a surgical maneuver over and over raises the odds of success when it matters. It is no different when preparing for an academic test. I was never in the upper half of my class in terms of innate intelligence. My IQ and the results of standardized testing were always pretty average. Yet, by working much harder than any of my classmates, I was able to graduate from college Phi Beta Kappa and later was elected into Alpha Omega Alpha, the highest honor society in medical school.

I agree with the saying that success is 1% inspiration and 99% perspiration. I believe that anyone can become an overachiever and attain his or her goals. Success is within the grasp of every individual who is willing to invest the time and effort necessary to be exquisitely well prepared.

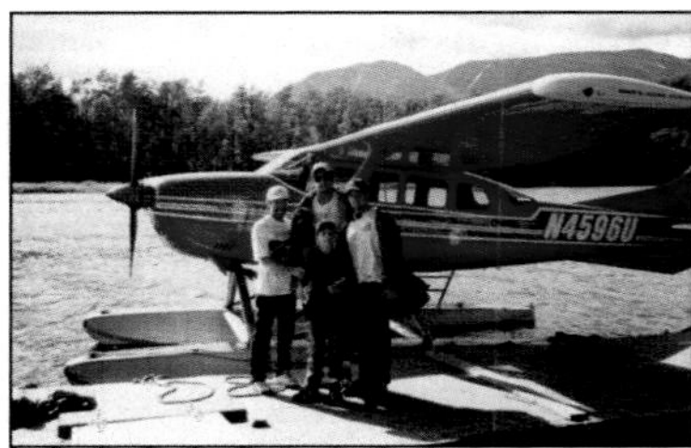

CHAPTER 4

Procrastination

Procrastination may not be evil enough to be among the sins listed in the Ten Commandments, but it sits atop the reasons why people with good intentions are ineffective. A general rule to live by might read, "If you think it should be done...then do it!" I can think of countless examples that underscore the importance of prompt execution, but none more poignant than the following incident. A few years ago, over the Thanksgiving holiday, one of my kids in college was enjoying a reunion with some of her high school friends at a large party. The sudden and unexpected arrival of a police officer unleashed a cascade of unfortunate events. The presence of open containers of beer led to a search, and a small bag of marijuana (when it was illegal) was discovered. Because my daughter happened to be in the closest proximity to the bag, she was cited for possession. I received a desperate phone call from my tearful child and, while she readily admitted to drinking beer, she denied having anything to do with the marijuana.

In a heartbeat, I told her to come home immediately, at which point I called a local hospital to find out if their laboratory was equipped to perform a complete drug screen. Fifteen minutes later, we were in the emergency department where she was urinating into a cup. Within 1 hour, I had incontestable proof that she was drug-free. I called the citing officer, and he acknowledged that he had not seen my daughter smoking the marijuana, but stated that she was the first to try to hide her beer! Furthermore, he admitted that the fresh aroma of marijuana was everywhere as the party was teeming with teenagers. At midnight, I called an attorney and explained the situation. To make a long story short, the negative drug screen turned out to be invaluable, and the drug possession charge was dropped. Her father was happy to pay both the attorney and the fine for an open container of alcohol.

Had I not acted promptly, the outcome might have been very different. While it was inconvenient to make a late-night trip to the emergency room, to procrastinate would probably have had serious consequences. She eventually became an outstanding nurse, but her admission to nursing school may have been in jeopardy. Our lives are filled with so many opportunities, many of which might be squandered if we allow our natural tendency to delay to prevail.

Osher RH. *The Real ABCs: A Surgeon's Analysis and a Father's Legacy, Second Edition* (pp 21-22).

I would suggest that the individual who wishes to become a high achiever take heed to the famous wedding quotation, "Speak now or forever hold your peace." Instead, your directive should become, "Act now or forever miss your moment!"

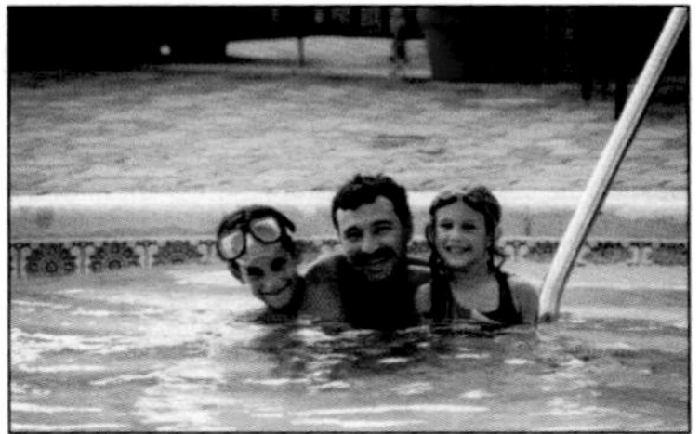

CHAPTER 5

Accepting the Challenge to Challenge the Accepted

I have heard a wide variety of terms used to describe my personality, some flattering and others not. If I had to make my own list, I would probably start with integrity and loyalty. Somewhere near the top, one might be surprised to find the word *renegade*. I am proud of the fact that I have spent much of my professional career challenging the status quo. While I do not believe that I am rebellious, I have never been able to accept the lame explanation, "because that's the way it is." Let me provide several specific examples.

When I enrolled at Trinity College in Hartford, Connecticut, I could not understand why the student snack bar closed several hours after dinner. It seemed to me that if students had to stay up late to study, then why not have easy access to a source of nourishment. Equally illogical was the fact that the athletic facilities would close so early. Why not leave the gym open to allow exercise in the evening? I brought these questions to the attention of a variety of administrators and could not even get a conversation started. As a result, I began campaigning to run for the College Council and was elected President by my fellow students. My first order of business was to keep the snack bar open until midnight and the gymnasium open until 10:00 pm (Figure 5-1). While my roommates were setting the political tone in the late 1960s by organizing rallies and protest marches, I was working up a sweat in the gym, followed by a delicious late-night snack!

During medical school, I was very interested in organizing a conference in a special field called *neuro-ophthalmology*, which did not exist at our hospital. I had won a 1-year-off fellowship award after finishing my first 2 years of the basic sciences, so I traveled to Miami, Florida to spend 12 months learning from a world-renowned neuro-ophthalmologist, J. Lawton Smith, MD (Figure 5-2). However, when I returned to the University of Rochester School of Medicine in New York, I was informed that third-year medical students were at the very bottom of the clinical totem pole, and our role was to *attend* rather than *organize* conferences. I went to the chairmen of the departments of ophthalmology and neurology and was able to convince Dr. Albert Snell, Jr. and Dr. Robert Joynt that I was worth a gamble. Within a short time, this monthly conference became one of the largest gatherings at the medical school. Who said it could not be done?

When I entered my residency in ophthalmology at the prestigious Bascom Palmer Eye Institute in Miami, I continued to challenge a variety of accepted practices. Because I often questioned the reasons behind medical decisions that seemed unfounded, a number of my teachers, as well as my peers, felt a bit threatened. In fact, at our annual resident's day skit, my cohorts projected an imaginary group photograph of the incoming residents intended to intimidate and

Osher RH. *The Real ABCs: A Surgeon's Analysis and a Father's Legacy, Second Edition* (pp 23-28).

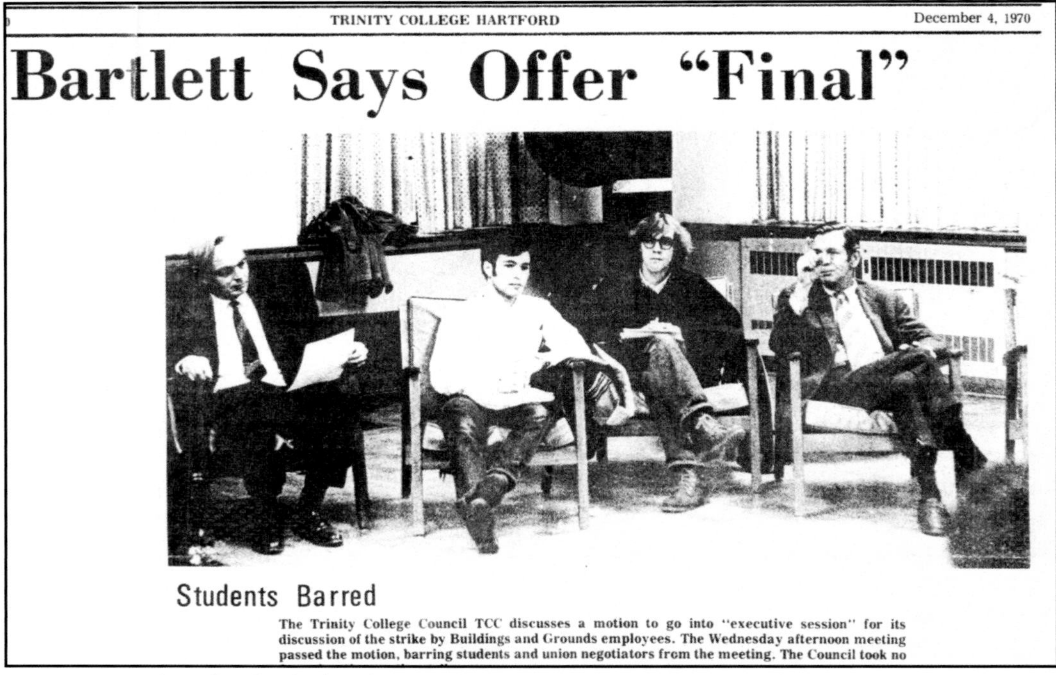

TRINITY COLLEGE HARTFORD December 4, 1970

Bartlett Says Offer "Final"

Students Barred

The Trinity College Council TCC discusses a motion to go into "executive session" for its discussion of the strike by Buildings and Grounds employees. The Wednesday afternoon meeting passed the motion, barring students and union negotiators from the meeting. The Council took no

Figure 5-1. President of student body, Bob Osher, demands an open gym and a late-night snack!

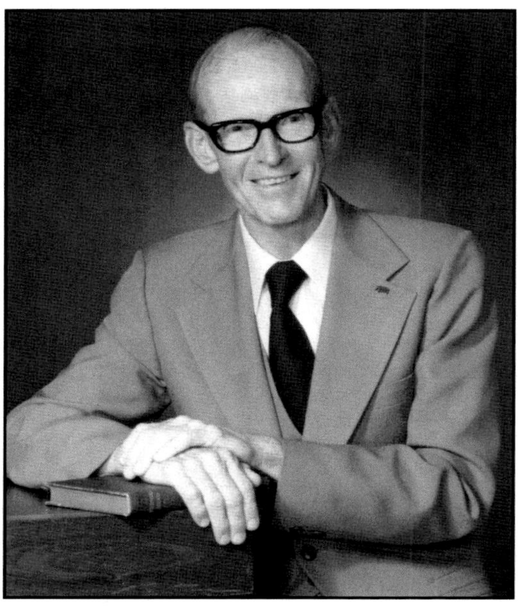

Figure 5-2. J. Lawton Smith, MD, renowned neuro-ophthalmologist at Bascom Palmer Eye Institute.

aggravate the faculty (Figure 5-3)! In my defense, I did develop wonderful relationships with the more secure individuals who reacted differently to my steady stream of challenges. I began to realize that most physicians do not like to be questioned, nor do they like change. People become comfortable with the status quo, especially in an environment like the operating room, where change creates stress. One might think that the medical profession would welcome innovation; unfortunately, the exact opposite is often true. I learned that almost every great innovator who changed ophthalmic surgery for the better was initially rejected and often tormented.

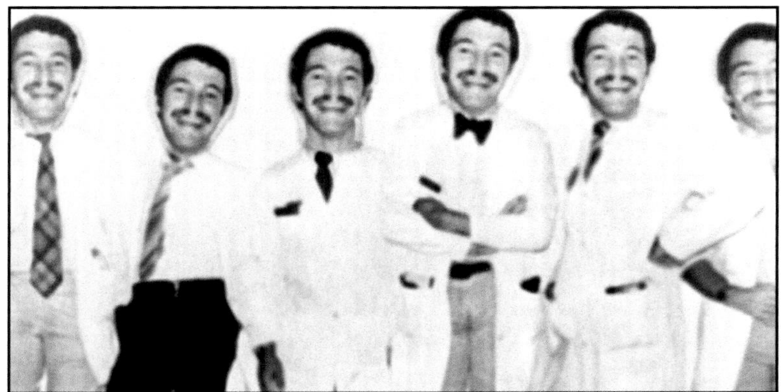

Figure 5-3. Faculty nightmare of incoming resident class.

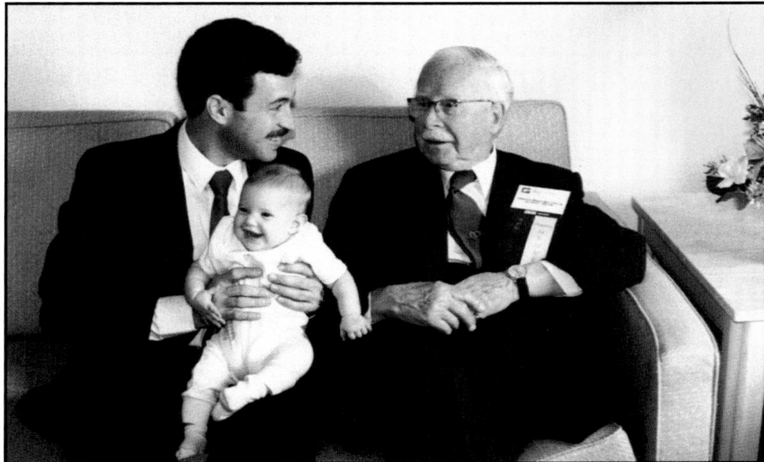

Figure 5-4. Sir Harold Riley, inventor of the intraocular lens, next to one of my babies, whom I helped to invent.

Sir Harold Ridley, the British ophthalmologist who truly improved mankind by developing the first intraocular lens used in conjunction with cataract surgery, was banished for the majority of his career (Figure 5-4). Just prior to his death, he was finally recognized and granted Knighthood by the Queen of England. Dr. Charles Kelman, just before he died, was inducted into the National Inventors' Hall of Fame for developing phacoemulsification, the elegant technique of removing a cataract through a microscopic incision. Instead of prolonged hospitalization and restricted activities, his brilliant concept allowed patients to undergo a far safer operation and return to a normal lifestyle immediately. Yet, in his book, *Through My Eyes*, one discovers that Dr. Kelman was severely ridiculed and scorned for years (Figure 5-5). Svyatoslav Fyodorov, MD, the Russian surgeon who pioneered the field of refractive surgery, was nearly exiled to Siberia, and his early disciples in the United States were ostracized (Figure 5-6). Many still believe that his premature death in a helicopter accident was not an accident! The list goes on in a sadly predictable fashion.

Early in my private practice, I was so lucky to have the support and counsel of my father, Dr. Morris Osher, a wonderful physician who was an early pioneer in the field of intraocular lens surgery. Even though he felt that I was somewhat overzealous in challenging the status quo, he always encouraged me to relentlessly pursue the truth. In the early 1980s, I introduced the first operation combining cataract surgery with astigmatism surgery and was the recipient of painful attacks from some of the foremost eye surgeons in the United States. I knew that the operation worked, but my efforts were met with disbelief and disparagement at every major meeting when

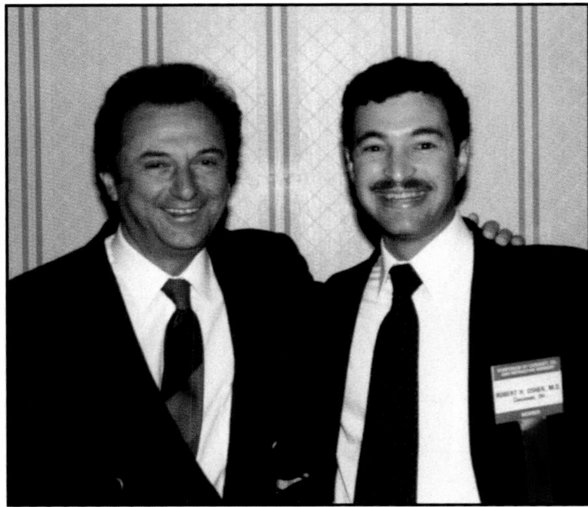

Figure 5-5. Dr. Charles Kelman, inventor of phacoemulsification.

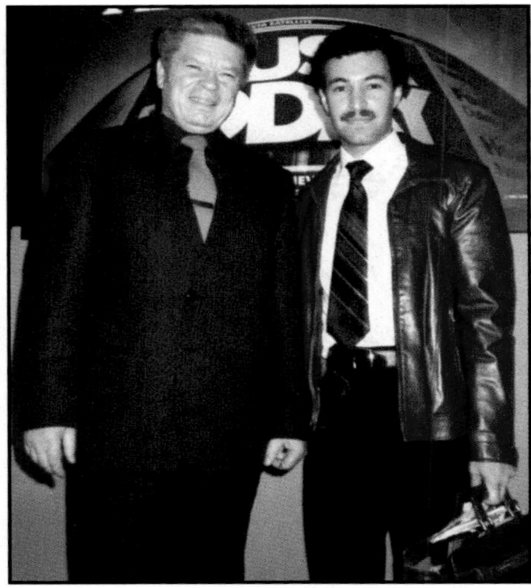

Figure 5-6. Dr. Svyatoslav Fyodorov, Russian pioneer in refractive surgery.

Figure 5-7. Mr. Peter Choyce, English implant pioneer writes a diplomatic letter.

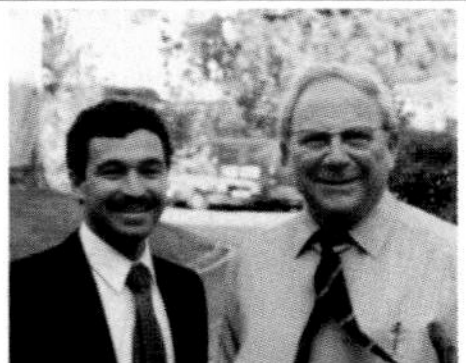

Robert H. Osher, M.D.
Cincinnati Eye Institute,
10494 Montgomery Road
Cincinnati, Ohio 45242, U.S.A.

Dear Bob,

I would appreciate a copy of the photograph which was taken in Guernsey.

You should run courses in how to stir up good controversy without giving offence!

See you soon I hope.

Yours sincerely,

Peter

18th October, 1986.

D.P. Choyce, MS, FRCS

I tried to discuss the technique and the positive results. In Europe, my work was so controversial that the response to my Keynote lecture in England was complete silence from the audience. The most famous eye surgeon at the meeting, Mr. Peter Choyce, sent me a letter of consolation with his understated English humor (Figure 5-7).

The same verbal assaults occurred when I performed the first clear lensectomy (removal of the transparent lens) for high hyperopia (extreme farsightedness) in 1986. Performing refractive surgery on a "normal eye" to correct thick glasses was so offensive to so many. Fortunately, Dr. J. Lawton Smith taught me that the truth is not defined by the majority opinion and cannot be suppressed indefinitely. Two decades later, I received the Nordan Lifetime Achievement Award and the Kelman Innovator's Award for advancing the field of refractive cataract surgery (Figure 5-8).

In the late 1980s, the Ioptex company introduced a new "surface passivated" intraocular lens that was alleged to have superior biologic properties. In order to avoid costly clinical studies, they asked the U.S. Food and Drug Administration for a regulatory exemption on the grounds that this lens was fundamentally the *same* as the standard intraocular lenses that were being

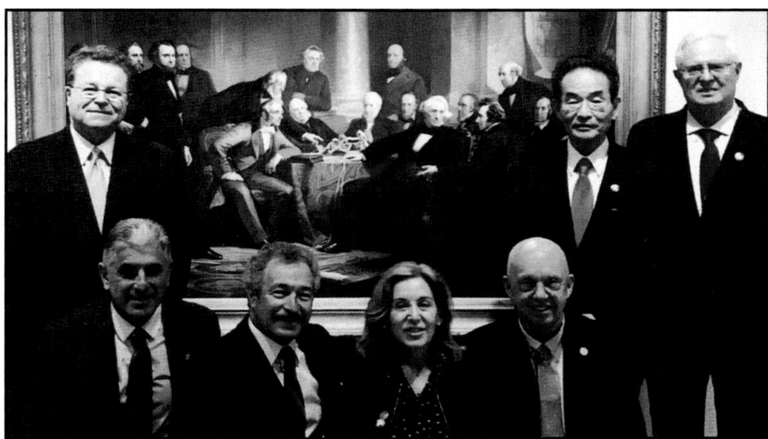

Figure 5-8. Innovator's Award recipients with Mrs. Ann Kelman by the famous, Men of Progress, National Portrait Gallery, Smithsonian Institute. (Reprinted with permission from David Chang, MD.)

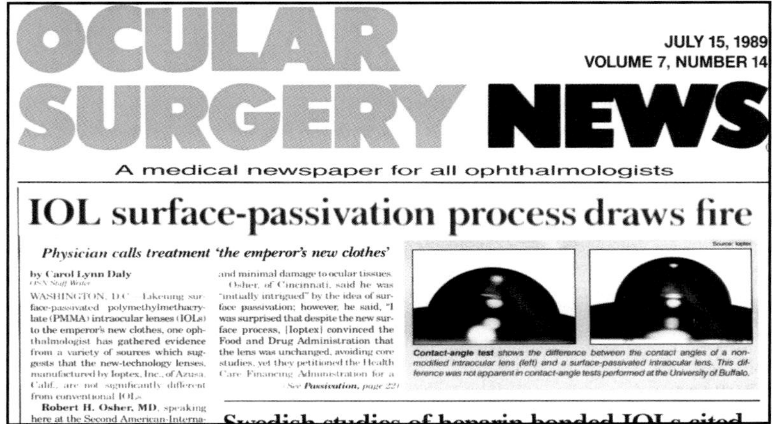

OCULAR SURGERY NEWS

JULY 15, 1989
VOLUME 7, NUMBER 14

A medical newspaper for all ophthalmologists

IOL surface-passivation process draws fire

Physician calls treatment 'the emperor's new clothes'

by Carol Lynn Daly
OSN Staff Writer

WASHINGTON, D.C.—Likening surface-passivated polymethylmethacrylate (PMMA) intraocular lenses (IOLs) to the emperor's new clothes, one ophthalmologist has gathered evidence from a variety of sources which suggests that the new-technology lenses, manufactured by Ioptex, Inc., of Azusa, Calif., are not significantly different from conventional IOLs.

Robert H. Osher, MD, speaking here at the Second American-Interna-

and minimal damage to ocular tissues.

Osher, of Cincinnati, said he was "initially intrigued" by the idea of surface passivation; however, he said, "I was surprised that despite the new surface process, [Ioptex] convinced the Food and Drug Administration that the lens was unchanged, avoiding core studies, yet they petitioned the Health Care Financing Administration for a

(See *Passivation*, page 22)

Source: Ioptex

Contact-angle test *shows the difference between the contact angles of a non-modified intraocular lens (left) and a surface-passivated intraocular lens. This difference was not apparent in contact-angle tests performed at the University of Buffalo.*

Swedish studies of heparin bonded IOLs cited

Figure 5-9. Attacked for exposing the truth about surface passivation.

implanted into the eyes of patients during routine cataract surgery. Yet, at the same time, Ioptex asked the Health Care Finance Administration, the government reimbursement agency, to allow an exorbitant fee of $450 per lens, alleging that this new process was dramatically *different* from the standard intraocular lenses. This contradiction reminded me of *Catch 22* by Joseph Heller. My suspicions were aroused, and after conducting studies performed by independent scientific laboratories, I was certain that this new process was analogous to sprinkling "pixie dust" onto the lens. The entire project was a hoax! The company must have heard about my investigation because they offered me a $50,000 consulting contract 2 weeks before the annual meeting of the American Society of Cataract and Refractive Surgery. I declined their offer! Then, at the Congress, following a series of presentations that made the lens sound miraculous, I stood up and presented my evidence, concluding that the Ioptex surface passivated intraocular lens was equivalent to the "emperor's new clothes." My presentation made the front page of the ophthalmic newspapers, drawing widespread criticism (Figure 5-9). Some of the most prominent leaders in cataract surgery were outraged and demanded that I make a public apology. However, I stood my ground, and within 1 year, the company had disappeared from the face of the earth.

Throughout my career, I have frequently questioned why we were performing cataract surgery the way we were and have often tried to develop methods of improving the most frequently performed operation in the United States. I was taught that phacoemulsification—the ultrasonic technique of removing a 10.5-mm cataract through a 3-mm incision—should not be performed

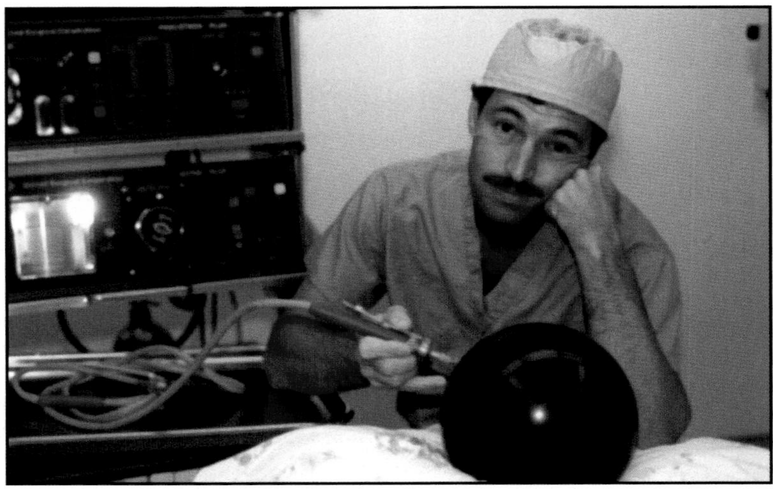

Figure 5-10. Developing a technique for emulsifying a "catarock."

when either the cataract was very hard (Figure 5-10), the pupil was small, the cornea was unhealthy, or the cataract was loose. I challenged each of these contraindications and developed new techniques that would offer our patients safer and better outcomes. The going was tough, and I was often called "dangerous" and "negligent" despite solid clinical evidence. Eventually, the critics began to vanish, and I gradually earned the respect of my colleagues through perseverance and hard work.

A video reviewing the controversial history and my role in the evolution of operating on the loose cataract just won an award at the Film Festival in Paris and received "Best of the Best" at the Annual Meeting of the American Academy of Ophthalmology in San Francisco.

Medicine is a profession where change consistently and predictably occurs. I like to tell our residents-in-training that today's dogma is tomorrow's dog poop! I encourage them to challenge the faculty and to make me defend my every maneuver or strategy in surgery. I believe that it is the obligation of every young surgeon to change ophthalmology, medicine, and the world for the better. Change is inevitable in everything in life; therefore, we should accept the challenge to challenge the accepted.

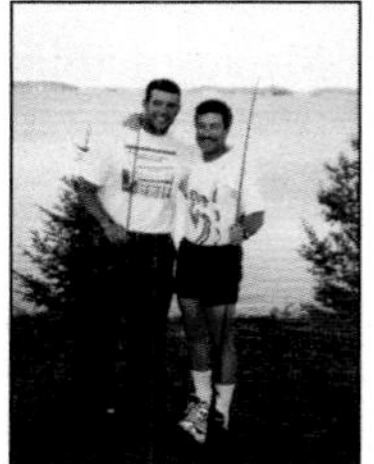

CHAPTER 6

Courage on the Cutting Edge

I never viewed myself as courageous. For that matter, I even have a problem with heights. Yet, I was quite surprised by my willingness to walk across the tightrope high above the comfort zone of the medical establishment when it came to evaluating cutting-edge technologies. Without a safety net below, the price for failure would be devastating—a loss of reputation for the surgeon and the possible loss of an eye for the patient.

Phacoemulsification is an amazing method of removing a cataract, developed by a New Yorker, Charles Kelman, MD. He stumbled upon the idea while in a dentist's chair, when he realized that the tiny ultrasonic drill might be used inside the eye. Traditionally, the cataract was removed in one piece by making a large incision about 12 mm in length. Dr. Kelman developed an ingenious system by which the lens could be broken up (emulsified) into tiny pieces by ultrasonic energy and removed through a 3-mm incision, an opening so small that sutures were not even required. Rather than suffering a long period of inactivity and slow visual recovery following hospitalization for large-incision cataract surgery, phacoemulsification allowed the patient to enjoy a rapid return to normal activities. Dr. Kelman's genius improved the lives and sight of many millions of patients around the world.

If there was a drawback to his technique, it was on the technical side. In the early days of phacoemulsification, these very complex and expensive machines offered only two options for vacuuming the pieces of the cataract: high and low. The high vacuum seemed unsafe since everything inside the eye happened with uncontrollable speed. By contrast, the low vacuum option was ineffective. It seemed so obvious to me that the surgeon needed to have infinite control of all variables inside the eye in order to provide the safest and most effective cataract operation. After approaching every American manufacturer and encountering one rejection after another, I began working with a small company in Italy and eventually developed a machine and a technique that I labeled "slow-motion" phacoemulsification (Figure 6-1). This method gave the surgeon exquisite control of events within the eye and allowed the surgeon to select a range of parameters never previously explored.

However, when I showed this technique to my teachers and to respected experts in the field of cataract surgery, they refused to believe that the "slow-motion" technique could work. I even developed a motorized intravenous pole to allow for the first time-adjustable, continuous infusion (Figure 6-2). Despite the lack of outside interest, I was certain that both this new technique and the technology of linear control represented an advance that eventually would allow the surgeon to select from an infinite range of variables, tailoring the operation to the individual patient. Slow-Motion Phacoemulsification allowed me to challenge the surgical contraindications

Osher RH. *The Real ABCs: A Surgeon's Analysis and a Father's Legacy, Second Edition* (pp 29-36).

Figure 6-1. Introducing slow-motion phacoemulsification with variable parameters, and Dr. Kelman's response.

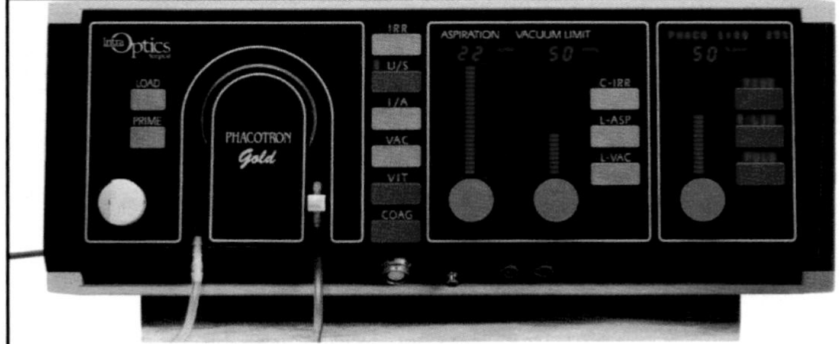

Dear Bob:

Thank you for responding to my request for an edited video of your surgical technique and accompanying commentary.

Your contribution regarding the technique of Slow Motion Phaco is highly important to phacoemulsification and I look forward to showing the videotape and crediting you for your achievement in this area.

With my thanks again and best wishes, I am

Sincerely yours,

Charles D. Kelman, M.D.

Figure 6-2. Automated intravenous pole introduces adjustable, continuous irrigation.

THE OSHER POWER IRRIGATION STAND

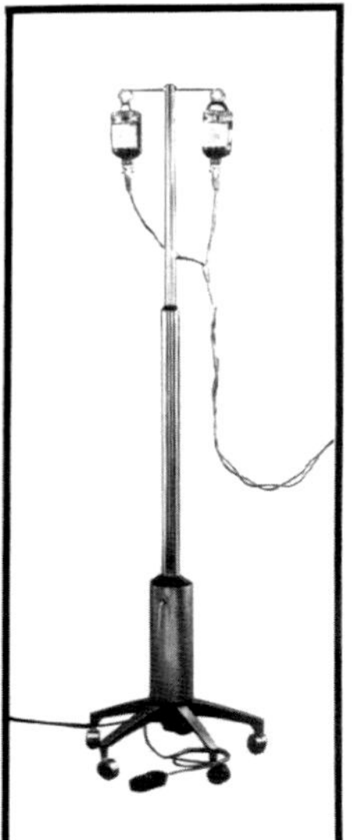

"For the Extra-Capsular Cataract Surgeon"

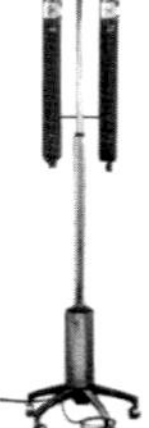

With the Osher Power Irrigation Stand, the surgeon is in control and will not have to delay while someone manually adjusts the IV stand. The power stand will provide fast and responsive adjustments of the IV bottle which can help reduce inundation of endothelial cells while maintaining the anterior chamber. It is far more stable than a regular IV stand, providing for a safer O.R.

The Osher Power Irrigation Stand is a motorized IV pole that is footswitch controlled. It has a travel of 29", starting at 57" from the floor to a maximum of 86".

The unit comes complete on a 5 castered base with foot control and power pack.

Catalog Number: 29-1750. **$1,495.00**

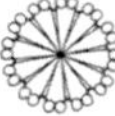

JEDMED INSTRUMENT COMPANY
1430 Hanley Industrial Court • St. Louis, MO 63144 • (314) 968-0822

A7-0110-84

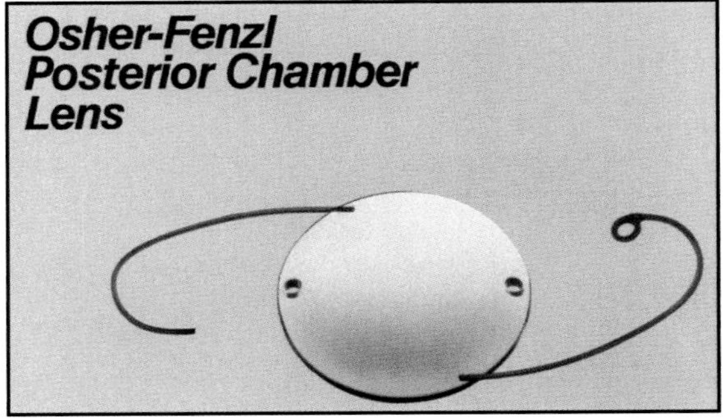

Figure 6-3. Osher-Fenzl intraocular lens.

established by Dr. Kelman, and I was able to operate on patients with loose cataracts, mature cataracts, compromised corneas, shallow chambers, and small pupils. I presented the initial series for using phacoemulsification in each of these taboo situations in the 1980s to skeptical audiences and, gradually, Slow-Motion Phacoemulsification drew the praise of colleagues around the planet. How ironic that it was Dr. Kelman's endorsement that officially validated my work (see Figure 6-1). These modifications have stood the test of time, and every contemporary machine offers these options today.

Marching to the beat of a different drum, I designed my first artificial lens implant with Johnson & Johnson during my first year of practice in 1981. The overwhelming majority of surgeons in the United States were placing the intraocular lens behind the iris in front of the capsular membrane in a location called the *ciliary sulcus*. Yet, God had located the human lens inside the capsular membranes, a place that seemed to be absolutely perfect. I felt so strongly about trying to duplicate our Creator's original design that I placed a small eyelet on the tip of the implant to help the surgeon insert the artificial lens into the original location of the natural lens within the sac or bag formed by the membranes. I believed in the benefits of this new design, and I stuck my neck out—in fact, way out—trying to convince the industry and my colleagues that this design by an unknown kid merited a huge financial investment to produce this implant. Within 1 to 2 years, the lens known as the *Osher-Fenzl lens* was being manufactured by each of the major companies and became one of the most popular designs in the United States. My entire reputation was linked to a device smaller than the size of a dime (Figure 6-3)!

At about the same time, I contacted two major companies, 3M and Surgikos, about designing a new protective eye drape to cover the lashes during surgery. Most surgeons would cut the eyelashes before surgery, but since the bacteria on the lids were still lurking next to the incision, I was convinced that a new drape design that completely covered the lids and lashes was necessary. I flew to Minneapolis, Minnesota and met with representatives of 3M, who rejected my idea on the spot. They advised me to stop wasting my time and to accept their top-selling fenestrated body drape that covered the entire patient. Surgikos, a division of Johnson & Johnson, had observed how well the Osher-Fenzl intraocular lens was doing, so they were willing to take a gamble. Within 1 year, their market share bypassed 3M into a leadership position. These small, transparent drapes that covered only the lids were accompanied by a wicking system, collection bag, and separate drape, which I designed to cover the machine. Ironically, this system, now manufactured by 3M, remains the standard of care today (Figure 6-4). In 2020, Beaver Visitec International will introduce a new concept in drape design that I have been working on for 3 years. The wheels of progress turn ever so slowly.

In the early 1990s, my fellow, Robert Cionni, MD, and I implanted the first capsular tension rings (CTR) in the United States. Loose cataracts resulting from either an injury or a birth defect were among the most difficult operations to perform. Surgeons in Japan and Germany had

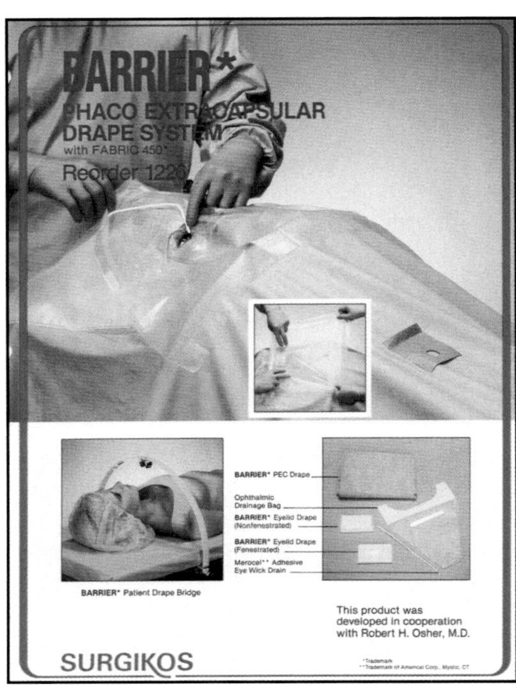

Figure 6-4. New draping system for eyelids and machine.

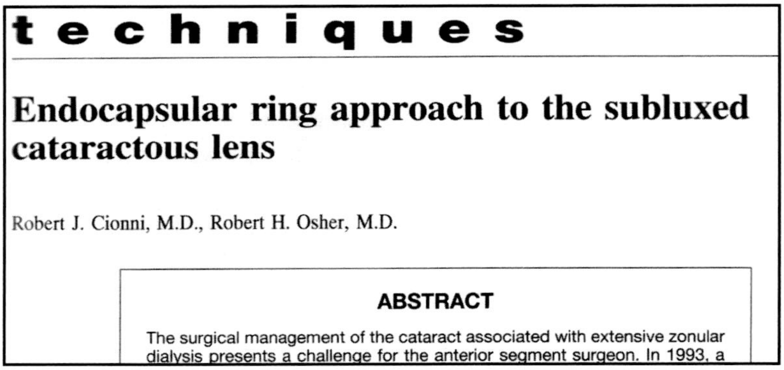

Figure 6-5. The CTR comes to America.

t e c h n i q u e s

Endocapsular ring approach to the subluxed cataractous lens

Robert J. Cionni, M.D., Robert H. Osher, M.D.

ABSTRACT

The surgical management of the cataract associated with extensive zonular dialysis presents a challenge for the anterior segment surgeon. In 1993, a

separately developed a device that behaved like a spring in the shape of a hula hoop, expanding the loose capsular bag. This spring would theoretically provide unprecedented stability and security for the intraocular lens in patients with a dangerously loose cataract. I was certain that this device could be a significant medical breakthrough for this unfortunate group of patients, so we began implanting the CTR in a small group of challenging cases and published the first series in the United States (Figure 6-5). I stood before members of the American Society of Cataract and Refractive Surgery presenting incredible results, and again, my reputation hung from a ring the size of a curled hair! At a large meeting in Chicago, Illinois, Dr. Manus Kraff, a famous cataract surgeon, announced to the audience that I was clearly engaging in medical malpractice. It required 11 years of battle, but the U.S. Food and Drug Administration (FDA) finally approved the device for human implantation in 2004, and it has become an essential surgical device. Dr. Cionni further modified the CTR, and his name is recognized by every cataract surgeon around the world.

The iris surrounds the pupil much like a doughnut surrounds the hole. It is the marvelous structure that opens and closes to regulate the amount of light entering the eye. Sadly, some individuals are either born without an iris or they lose the iris as a result of a tragic accident.

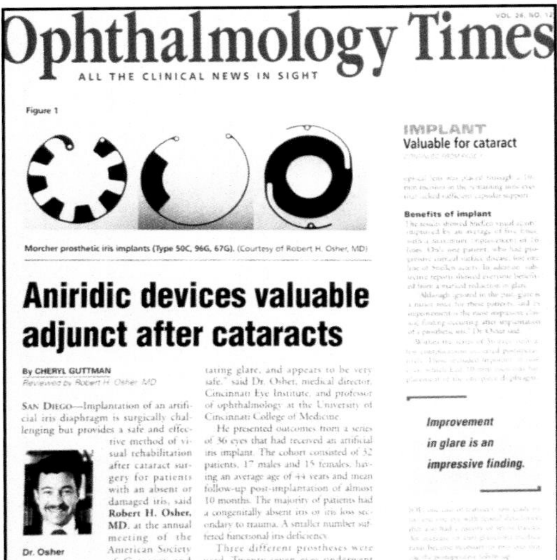

Ophthalmology Times

ALL THE CLINICAL NEWS IN SIGHT

Figure 1

Morcher prosthetic iris implants (Type 50C, 96G, 67G). (Courtesy of Robert H. Osher, MD)

Aniridic devices valuable adjunct after cataracts

By CHERYL GUTTMAN

Reviewed by Robert H. Osher, MD

SAN DIEGO—Implantation of an artificial iris diaphragm is surgically challenging but provides a safe and effective method of visual rehabilitation after cataract surgery for patients with an absent or damaged iris, said **Robert H. Osher, MD**, at the annual meeting of the American Society of Cataract and

Dr. Osher

tating glare, and appears to be very safe," said Dr. Osher, medical director, Cincinnati Eye Institute, and professor of ophthalmology at the University of Cincinnati College of Medicine.

He presented outcomes from a series of 36 eyes that had received an artificial iris implant. The cohort consisted of 32 patients, 17 males and 15 females, having an average age of 44 years and mean follow-up post-implantation of almost 10 months. The majority of patients had a congenitally absent iris or iris loss secondary to trauma. A smaller number suffered functional iris deficiency.

Three different prostheses were used. Twenty-seven eyes underwent

IMPLANT

Valuable for cataract

Benefits of implant

Improvement in glare is an impressive finding.

Figure 6-6. Our experience with the artificial iris. The first American series.

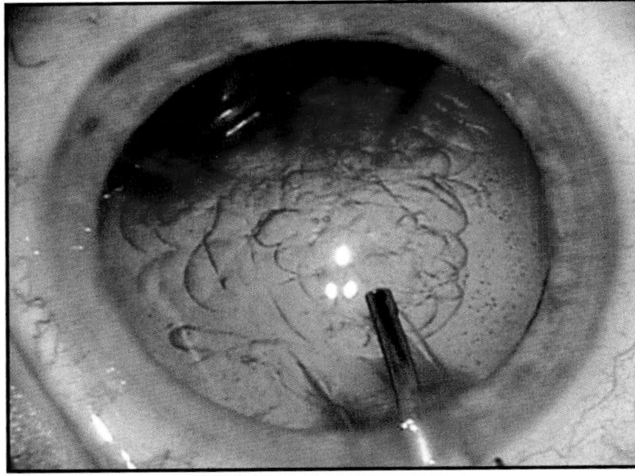

Figure 6-7. HEALON5 injected into the eye.

Mr. Peter Choyce, the English surgeon mentioned in Chapter 5, developed the first artificial iris in 1956, but the idea was abandoned. When German surgeons developed a more modern artificial iris device, Ken Rosenthal, MD from New York brought the idea to the United States in 1996. Based on his pioneering case, I became the first American surgeon to use a partial prosthesis as well as the artificial iris containing an intraocular lens, publishing the initial series of patients in which a dramatic reduction in glare was documented (Figure 6-6). Within months after the article appeared, patients were being referred from as far away as Maine and Alaska for artificial iris implantation. I did not care that not a single insurance company would cover this procedure, and I often bought these expensive devices from European companies and performed the surgery for my patients free of charge. I was, however, very concerned about risking my medical license as well as my financial nest egg by undertaking a procedure not approved in the United States. One unexpected complication could mean that a malpractice suit might end my career. Yet, if a surgeon wants to explore the cutting edge of technology, he or she must be prepared to shoulder the unknown risks and possible consequences. I followed the advice of Douglas Koch, MD, the President of the American Cataract Society, who insisted that I protect myself by notifying the FDA of my early work. Joined by several of my conscientious partners (Scott Burk, MD, PhD; Michael Snyder, MD; and Edward Holland, MD), our institution has performed more of these operations than anywhere in the United States. Twenty-one years later, the prosthetic iris finally received FDA approval.

When it comes to bringing my patients the best possible technology, I have always been willing to take some political and regulatory gambles. For example, HEALON5 (Johnson & Johnson) is a jelly-like lubricant that is injected into the eye to protect all of the delicate structures like the cornea during surgery (Figure 6-7). It also prevents the eye from collapsing like an airless balloon once an incision has been made. I was aware that this product was being developed in Sweden, so I began "smuggling" it into the country for the benefit of my patients before anyone in America knew about it, 4 long years before it was approved by the FDA. Dozens of patients with severe corneal disease who could not have undergone cataract surgery without a simultaneous corneal transplant were able to avoid this major operation because of HEALON5.

My unauthorized use of a capsular dye is another example of challenging the standard of care. Rarely, a patient neglects the cataract for such a long period of time that it turns as white

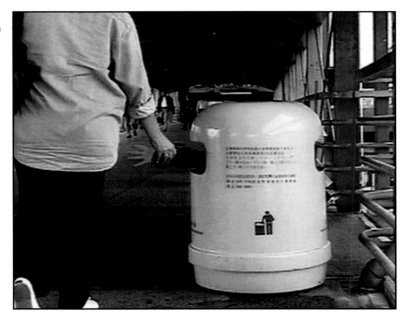

Figure 6-8. I wish medical school had offered a course in smuggling.

as a snowball. It is very difficult to operate on this type of cataract because the clear membranes become invisible against the white background. A surgeon from the Netherlands and another surgeon from Japan independently introduced a technique for staining the membranes with an inky substance, which is generically called a *capsular dye*. Its color makes the operation far safer for the patient. Unfortunately, the FDA decided to classify this dye as a drug, which meant a costly and prolonged approval procedure. Rather than encounter the increased likelihood of significant complications when trying to remove a white cataract, I used the dye for almost 7 years before it was approved by the FDA and our results were published. While I never felt at ease smuggling in these products (Figure 6-8), I was certain that placing patient benefit above personal risk was justified.

It has been both frightening and exhilarating to be the first surgeon to use a new device in the United States. I've encountered a patient with a blind eye and a cataract so white it could be seen across the room with the naked eye. Implanting a solid black intraocular lens resulted in a patient so happy with her cosmetic appearance that she cried tears of joy, despite having no sight in the operated eye (Figure 6-9). I also implanted the first small aperture lens, a solid lens with a tiny peep hole in the middle, developed by Brazilian surgeon, Dr. Claudio Trindade. My initial patient was a schoolteacher who had undergone multiple radial keratotomy surgeries elsewhere that left her with so much astigmatism and glare that she was confined to her home. This surgery resulted in a patient thrilled with her excellent vision and near absence of incapacitating glare (Figure 6-10). I've even published a series of patients who had longstanding, stable, double vision in whom I implanted a lens for distance in one eye and a very strong lens for near in the fellow eye, an operation I called *Intentional Extreme Pseudophakic Monovision* (Figure 6-11). The result was a delighted group of patients who could see both at a distance and very close without glasses. Best of all, the double vision was gone! Boy, did this create controversy, but this operation was a new cure for double vision.

Finally, I have always believed that size matters when it comes to incision length: the smaller, the better, as long as quality is not compromised. In 2005, I was privileged to work with Val Injev, PE, MBA, a scientist from Alcon. Together we "pushed the envelope," introducing a new procedure for removing the cataract through a 2.2-mm opening, an operation we called *microcoaxial*

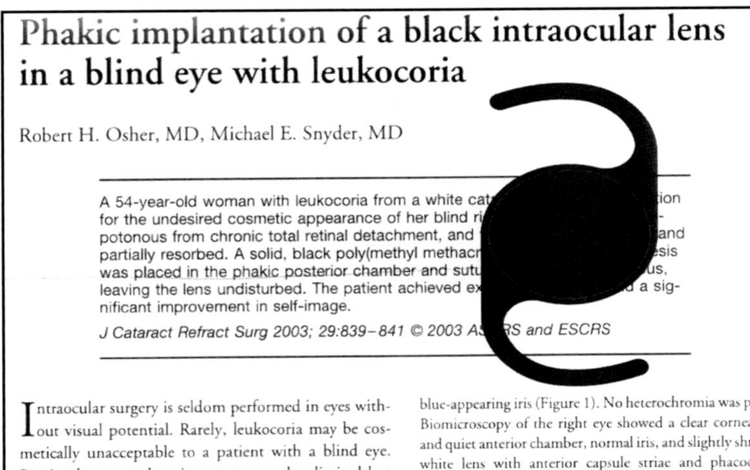

Phakic implantation of a black intraocular lens in a blind eye with leukocoria

Robert H. Osher, MD, Michael E. Snyder, MD

A 54-year-old woman with leukocoria from a white cat ion for the undesired cosmetic appearance of her blind ri - potonous from chronic total retinal detachment, and and partially resorbed. A solid, black poly(methyl methacr sis was placed in the phakic posterior chamber and sutu us, leaving the lens undisturbed. The patient achieved e a significant improvement in self-image.

J Cataract Refract Surg 2003; 29:839–841 © 2003 A S and ESCRS

Intraocular surgery is seldom performed in eyes without visual potential. Rarely, leukocoria may be cosmetically unacceptable to a patient with a blind eye. Previously reported options are somewhat limited but

blue-appearing iris (Figure 1). No heterochromia was pre Biomicroscopy of the right eye showed a clear cornea, and quiet anterior chamber, normal iris, and slightly shru white lens with anterior capsule striae and phacodo

Figure 6-9. Solid Black IOL—Morcher Type 80D, which I have used to attain excellent cosmesis in a patient with severe leukocoria in a blind, hypotonous eye that we published in the peer-reviewed literature.

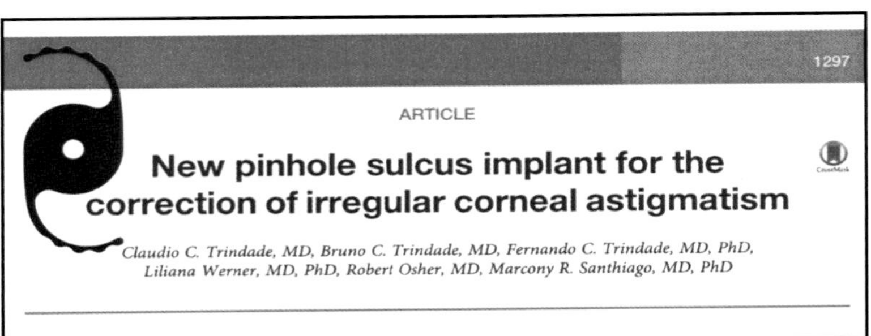

1297

ARTICLE

New pinhole sulcus implant for the correction of irregular corneal astigmatism

Claudio C. Trindade, MD, Bruno C. Trindade, MD, Fernando C. Trindade, MD, PhD, Liliana Werner, MD, PhD, Robert Osher, MD, Marcony R. Santhiago, MD, PhD

Figure 6-10. Small Aperture IOL. Designed by Brazilian surgeon, Claudio Trindade, MD, this small aperture IOL (Morcher Type 93L) has proven to be a brilliant innovation in patients with irregular corneal astigmatism due to radial keratotomy, keratoconus, and previous trauma. Patients with intractable glare also attained relief in our peer-reviewed publication.

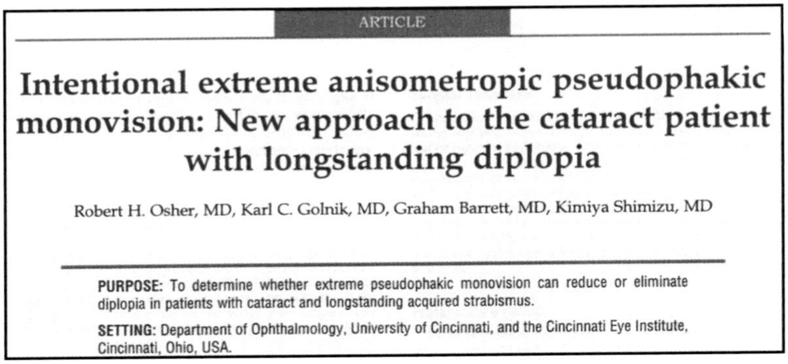

ARTICLE

Intentional extreme anisometropic pseudophakic monovision: New approach to the cataract patient with longstanding diplopia

Robert H. Osher, MD, Karl C. Golnik, MD, Graham Barrett, MD, Kimiya Shimizu, MD

PURPOSE: To determine whether extreme pseudophakic monovision can reduce or eliminate diplopia in patients with cataract and longstanding acquired strabismus.

SETTING: Department of Ophthalmology, University of Cincinnati, and the Cincinnati Eye Institute, Cincinnati, Ohio, USA.

Figure 6-11. A new cure for patients with stable, long-standing, double vision using two intraocular lenses: one targeted for distance and the other implanted for very close vision. The peer-reviewed publication generated lots of controversy.

phacoemulsification. By reducing the incision size more than 25%, the procedure was even safer and with less postoperative-induced astigmatism. We published a two-part article in the *Journal of Cataract & Refractive Surgery* in 2007, in which we reported our laboratory and my initial clinical results (Figure 6-12). It was not easy figuring out how to get a 13.5-mm intraocular lens with a 6-mm optic into the eye through a 2.2-mm incision. We had to modify the configuration of the incision, developing an "internal flare," which was initially rejected by every American journal (so I knew that it must be really good). Eventually, this new incision was published, and microcoaxial phacoemulsification, still the standard of care in the United States, was selected as a milestone achievement during the 50-year celebration of phacoemulsification organized by the American Society of Cataract and Refractive Surgery (Figure 6-13).

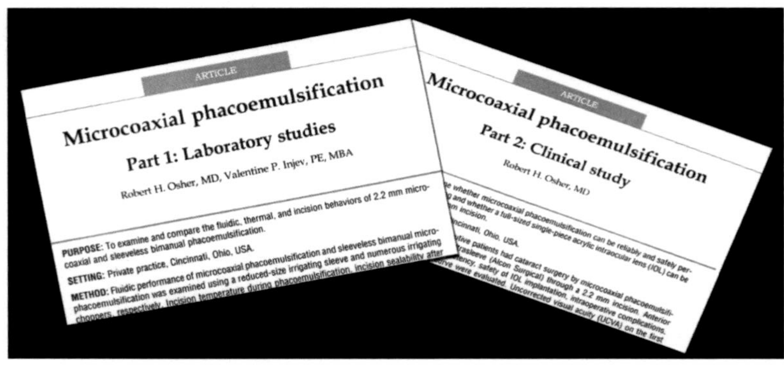

ARTICLE

Microcoaxial phacoemulsification

Part 1: Laboratory studies

Robert H. Osher, MD, Valentine P. Injev, PE, MBA

PURPOSE: To examine and compare the fluidic, thermal, and incision behaviors of 2.2 mm micro-coaxial and sleeveless bimanual phacoemulsification.

SETTING: Private practice, Cincinnati, Ohio, USA.

METHOD: Fluidic performance of microcoaxial phacoemulsification and sleeveless bimanual micro-phacoemulsification was examined using a reduced-size irrigating sleeve and numerous irrigating choppers, respectively. Incision temperature during phacoemulsification, incision sealability after

ARTICLE

Microcoaxial phacoemulsification

Part 2: Clinical study

Robert H. Osher, MD

Figure 6-12. Size matters: microcoaxial phacoemulsification is introduced in 2007 and remains the standard of care in the United States.

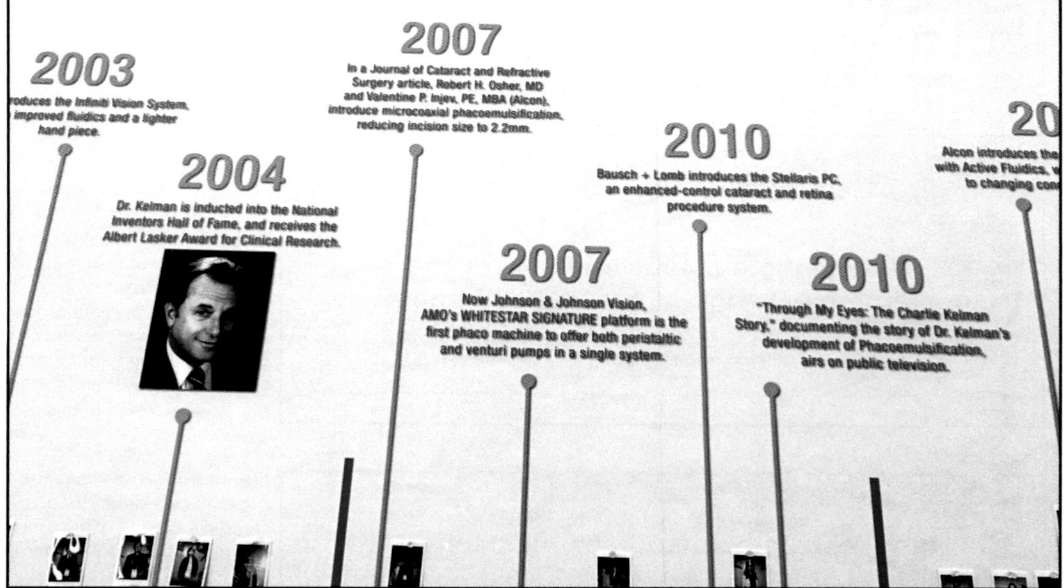

Figure 6-13. Our contribution was recognized on the Timeline of Milestones exhibited at 50-Year Celebration in Washington, DC.

Presenting my surgical experience at scientific meetings and publishing my results has been a slow but effective way to change the standard of care in the medical profession. Sometimes, it is necessary to take a lonely position "outside the box," where one is neither comfortable nor completely safe. Under these circumstances, a little bit of courage and a lot of conviction goes a long way.

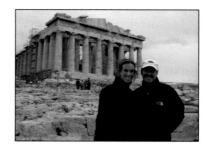

CHAPTER 7

Time Management

There is so little time to get everything done that one would like to accomplish in a given day, week, month, or even during a lifetime. I have tried to explain to my children that the hardest task in time management is the act of getting started. There are mental and physical landmines everywhere as there is always some distraction or opportunity to procrastinate. With hundreds of television channels to watch and the internet to surf, one could waste 24 hours each day, sitting mesmerized in front of some screen. Nothing would ever get done! I was so happy when our large screen television exploded. Instantly, my children were freed from the couch, where they had become imprisoned zombies. Now, years later, I just have to once again figure out how to sabotage my grandchildren's computer games and cell phones!

If one wants to achieve something, there must be a plan in place, and the time requirements must be realistic and then respected. In other words, a project must be assigned an appropriate amount of time, along with a schedule that will permit the task to be initiated and then completed, but not necessarily at the same sitting. Every evening, I always make a list of the top-priority items that must be accomplished the next day. Between traffic lights, operations, or patient appointments, I will attack this list one item at a time, and by the end of the day, it is remarkable how many things have been completed. To procrastinate is human, but the high achiever is constantly trying to knock off as many chores, responsibilities, and projects as possible.

An important principle is to avoid allowing too much to accumulate on the "back burner." The amount of work either becomes intimidating or stuff just gets overlooked and forgotten. There is truth to the maxim that states, "if you want something done, give the task to the person who is always the busiest." He or she is used to prioritizing and multitasking and will find a way to get it done!

Another invaluable lesson is that incremental volumes of work accomplished during multiple settings add up to something big. I call this strategy *aliquot planning*. In chemistry, an aliquot represents a small unit. Aliquot planning means that a large project can be achieved by working in small aliquots. In other words, to write a thesis, one cannot enter the library at 8:00 pm and emerge at midnight with a completed first-class manuscript. It requires many sessions where the cumulative effect of small aliquots of effort is the finished project. For example, if one cleans a portion of a closet every day, by the end of the week, an onerous, unpleasant job is more likely to have been successfully completed. Writing this book is another good example. It has taken many months of work, often one thought or topic at a time, but when the individual paragraphs were arranged into chapters and the chapters were linked together, the cumulative result was a book.

Osher RH. *The Real ABCs: A Surgeon's Analysis and a Father's Legacy, Second Edition* (pp 37-39).

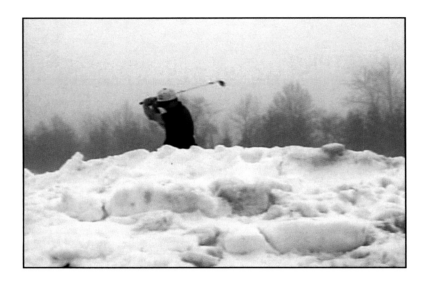

Figure 7-1. Year-round practice makes perfect!

It is remarkable just how much can be achieved through the summation of multiple work sessions. I was able to teach myself to speak Portuguese by ordering 30 introductory tapes, 30 intermediate tapes, and then 30 advanced tapes. Every time I was driving to some destination, I simply listened to a portion of a tape rather than indulge in some non-productive radio chatter. While nothing could be achieved in a single day, week, or even month, over the course of 1 year, I learned to "falo Portuguese."

I utilized the same strategy to teach myself to play golf. I practiced a little bit every day, one session with my driver, another on my irons, another in the bunkers, then chipping or pitching or putting…over and over again, year-round (Figure 7-1). The repetition was combined with extensive reading. The result was that I could shoot in the 80s by the end of my first year and in the 70s by the close of year 2! The same logic applies to planting a garden, writing a manuscript, learning to play a sport, or mastering a job-related goal.

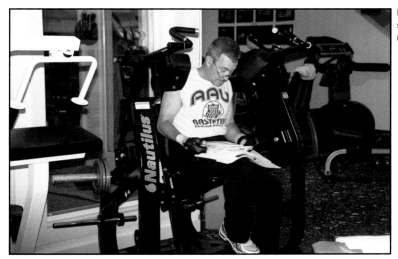

Figure 7-2. Time management survival strategy—opening mail between exercises.

There are other tricks that will help facilitate getting things done. Multitasking is a strategy that makes good sense. When I lift weights and need to rest for a few minutes between exercises, I will spend this time wisely by keeping my briefcase at my side so I can open my mail (Figure 7-2). When my wife and I are going somewhere, I will ask her to take the wheel so that I can work on my surgery charts while she drives. Between patients in the office, my secretary still hands me printed copies of emails to read, prioritize, answer, or discard. During my short lunch break, I try to get through several telephone calls. On an airplane, while most passengers are watching a movie, I prefer to use this uninterrupted time to work on a manuscript or to plan upcoming surgeries since I always have access to my medical records when traveling.

While everyone needs a little do nothing "down time" to recharge our batteries, I am convinced that the efficient utilization of time is a key ingredient in achieving our potential and allowing us to enjoy a full and meaningful life.

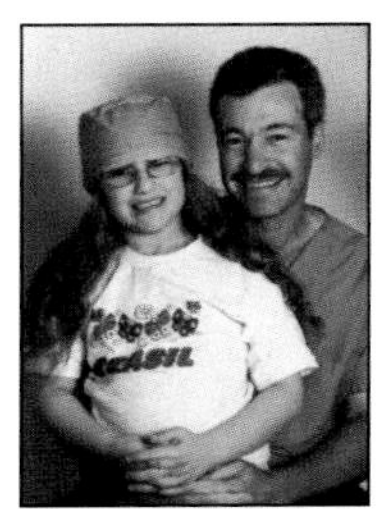

CHAPTER 8

Mistake Management

I have built my reputation in the field of cataract surgery by showing how to manage the complications that every surgeon encounters. What has been unique is that I have paraded my own difficulties and even my mistakes in front of colleagues for their educational benefit. In doing so, I have learned an important lesson: to err is human.* Yet, it is equally human to attempt to cover-up or deny fault. Each of us would like to be recognized for our competency and, therefore, a less-than-ideal result seems to threaten our self-esteem or, perhaps, compromise the respect that we would like to receive from others.

In my opinion, it takes considerable strength to acknowledge that an error has been made. There is truth to the George Washington fable where a candid admission of guilt turns out to be the best solution. Most of the time, the one who committed the offense may still be in hot water, but the temperature is turned down several degrees following a sincere apology. I recently heard about a medical school in which the physicians were being taught how to apologize to patients in an effort to reduce malpractice litigation. I am confident that it would have turned out much differently for slick Bill Clinton or Tiger Woods had each simply said, "I'm sorry" with genuine sincerity. I am still apologizing to my ex-wife for being a lousy husband, and our relationship today is warm and supporting as we work together to keep our family strong.

Why is this discussion relevant? When one is determined to achieve, he or she is more likely to inadvertently trounce on someone's feelings or to commit an insensitive act. While Achievement is not incompatible with thoughtfulness and sensitivity, the typical achiever is often intensely focused or too preoccupied to recognize his or her transgression. I am sure that I have offended my staff by being abrupt when I am behind in the clinic, my family by charging at some goal "come hell or high water," and my colleagues by wasting little time to consider diplomacy when challenging a presentation. The best mistake management that I have learned is to offer a sincere apology, then to express my intention to do better. After a while, it becomes very easy to say, "I made a mistake and I am sorry," rather than becoming defensive or denying wrongdoing.

The mistakes that have hurt me the most are the ones related to my family, which, unfortunately, I was too blind to see at the time. I really thought that I was a pretty good father. I coached all of the teams, went to all of the plays and recitals, told bedtime stories, took the kids trick-or-treating, and paid for an excellent education for each of my children. However, in the eyes of a youngster, these acts do not even register. Only now, when my children are grown up,

* Alexander Pope, *Essay on Criticism*, 1711

am I learning just how many terrible mistakes I had made. My past insensitivity causes my heart to ache. How I wish I could retract casual statements related to weight or appearance that were said for a positive reason but completely backfired. I learned everything in medical school, but failed the domestic IQ test.

Now, as I turn age 70, I am learning that being a parent is much more than providing a home, an education, discipline, rewards for good behavior, an annual vacation, a new ball glove, and a nice bike. Children need, more than anything else, a sense of security in knowing that they are deeply loved and respected. How I wish life had a reverse button and I could do it all over. This time, I would pay less attention to achieving my own goals and more attention to their feelings. I would say, "I'm sorry that I accidentally hurt your feelings; I love you." "No, you can't color on the wall or tell a lie or eat candy between meals." Then, I would add, "But I'm the luckiest father in the world to have you as a son or daughter. You're beautiful inside and out and I'll always be there for you. You make me so proud!" For missing the opportunity to empathize and to apologize then, I am still apologizing now.

It is a given that the optimal approach for every high achiever would be to avoid making mistakes and to be hypersensitive to the feelings of family and coworkers. However, since most goal-oriented individuals are focused on Achievement and are more likely to upset somebody, a quick and sincere apology for the insensitivity or miscue remains the best mistake management. Don't wait! The sooner one learns this difficult career and domestic lesson, the happier he or she will be as an achiever and as a person.

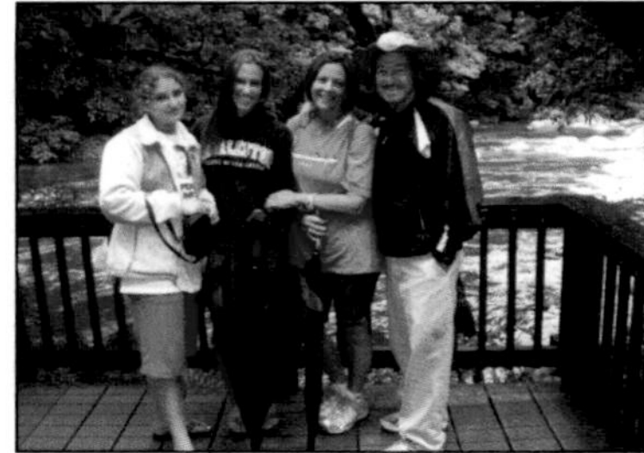

CHAPTER 9

Fitness

There really is something to the old saying, "sound body and sound mind." One must designate time for fitness in order to achieve Balance and a sense of well-being. Granted, after a long day at work, it is often very difficult to initiate an exercise program, especially if you are exhausted and have to travel to a distant gym. However, just as discipline is required for professional achievement, it is also required in order to stay physically fit.

The human body is a compilation of miracle after miracle. As an ophthalmologist, I am still in awe over the complex neuroanatomic pathways that make the gift of sight possible. Yet, miracles aside, if the body is neglected, bad things happen. It is alarming how quickly one can get out of shape and gain weight. Fortunately, it is equally amazing how the human body can recover by shedding pounds, gaining muscle, and improving endurance. I believe it is a fallacy that one can get back into shape like flipping a light switch whenever he or she wishes. Another fallacy is that the purchase of expensive exercise equipment by itself will get the job done. In order to get fit and stay fit, exercise has to be a way of life, just like eating and sleeping. It does not take much time to get a good workout, usually less than the time one wastes in pondering when and where to exercise.

The rewards of staying fit are enormous: when one looks healthy and in shape, one feels good. When one feels good, things tend to get done and Achievement may come easier. Unfortunately, the majority of people have difficulty achieving their goals in life the same way the majority are unable to stay fit. The reason is ridiculously simple…it is tough! My friend, Mark Becker, who owns an exercise equipment store, tells me that, just after New Year's Day, his sales skyrocket because everyone makes a resolution to get fit. However, after several months, he has found that recently purchased exercise equipment is usually collecting cobwebs or serving as an expensive clothes hanger.

I began running more than 50 years ago in college, long before running became fashionable (Figure 9-1). After classes, I would run for 30 minutes, take a shower, and then I was ready to hit the books. In medical school, after an evening of intense study, I would always go to the gym before midnight to work up a good sweat. At age 60, I had to give up running as years of playing tennis and running on asphalt in lousy shoes had taken a toll on my knees. However, biking, kayaking, swimming, and lifting weights have been sufficient to maintain my mental health and physical well-being (Figure 9-2). Following my nephrectomy, I was only able to do a handful of push-ups, but 1 year later, I was able to knock off 100 as a result of the remarkable capability of the human body (Figure 9-3). As I turn age 70, I cannot hit the numbers that I used to crunch, but I am still trying to push myself almost every day after work. When I think of money well

Osher RH. *The Real ABCs: A Surgeon's Analysis and a Father's Legacy, Second Edition* (pp 43-44).

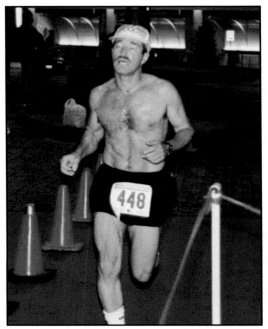

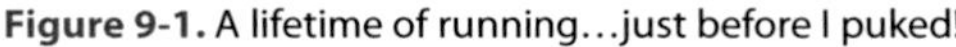
Figure 9-1. A lifetime of running…just before I puked!

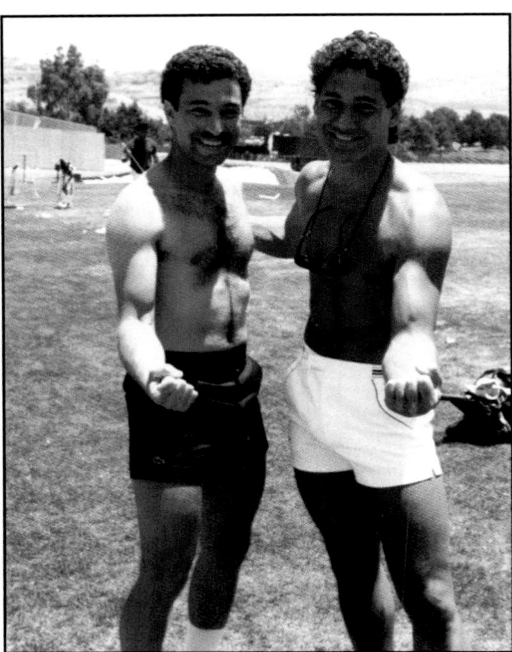

Figure 9-2. Who is the Olympian: Osher or Louganis?

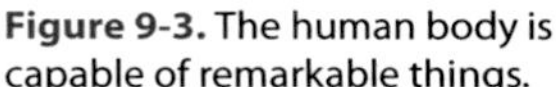
Figure 9-3. The human body is capable of remarkable things.

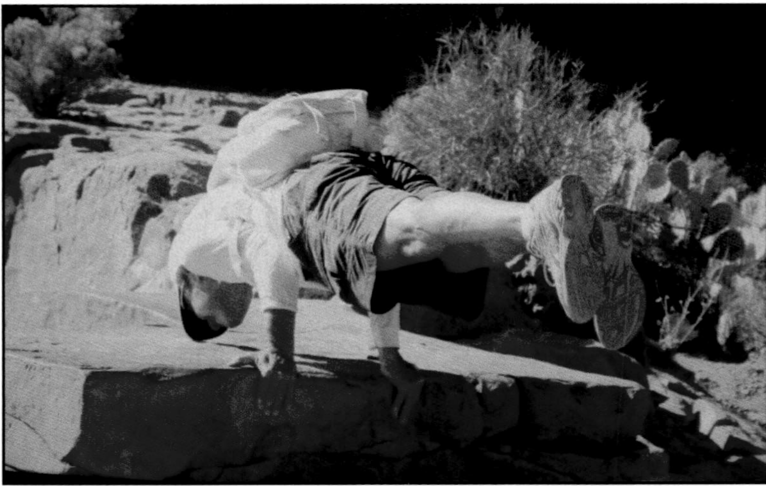

spent, either joining a health club or hiring a trainer and then really taking exercise seriously has to be one of life's best investments.

The lesson here is simple and best stated by the Nike maxim: "Just do it." One will never regret being in shape!

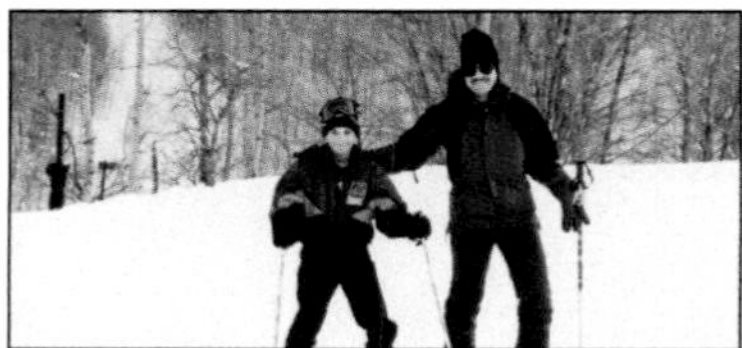

CHAPTER 10

Critical Balance

The Ratio of Hard Work to Hard Play

Understanding the concept of Balance is an essential key to a meaningful life that is marked by Achievement. I believe that too much of anything will cause desensitization to even the most pleasurable events and activities. This includes chocolate, money, sex, etc. In medicine, there is a term called *tachyphylaxis*, which means that the initial effect will begin to diminish over time. For example, a glaucoma medication may initially reduce the pressure inside the eye by 50%, but eventually, it begins to lose some of its potency. How good does that first bite of your favorite dessert taste? Then, after several bites, the taste buds become saturated by the sweet stimulus, and then the blood sugar begins to rise, at which point the delicious flavor decreases. Over a prolonged period of time, overindulgence produces diminishing returns. A personal example applies to my childhood favorite dessert, blueberry pie. When I was a youngster, I could barely wait for dinnertime because I knew that my mother always had a seemingly endless supply of blueberry pie. However, after months and months of blueberry pie, not only did I cease to enjoy this dessert, but I have never had any interest in ordering it during the past 6 decades!

Hence, the concept of Balance. If one is going to achieve, it is necessary to work very hard. However, it is equally necessary to get away from work and to also play very hard. Then, it becomes possible to resume the work-related task with efficiency and renewed enthusiasm. I always have attempted to set a time limit on just how long I would work, knowing that there was a reward such as exercise, a pizza, or something representing a light at the end of the tunnel. Even in medical school where hours upon hours of study were necessary, I never failed to schedule some recreational activity during the course of an onerous evening. At about 11:00 pm, I would sprint to the hospital gym, turn on the lights, and shoot baskets or exercise for 1 hour. Refreshed, I could resume working and stay focused for a while longer.

Osher RH. *The Real ABCs: A Surgeon's Analysis and a Father's Legacy, Second Edition* (pp 45-46).

Having the discipline to string numerous work sessions together interspersed with scheduled playtime to recharge your mental battery is a highly effective strategy that eventually gets lots of big jobs done. Learning to undertake and organize multiple projects simultaneously, and balancing hard work, recreation, and fitness gives you access to the passing lane on the Road to Achievement.

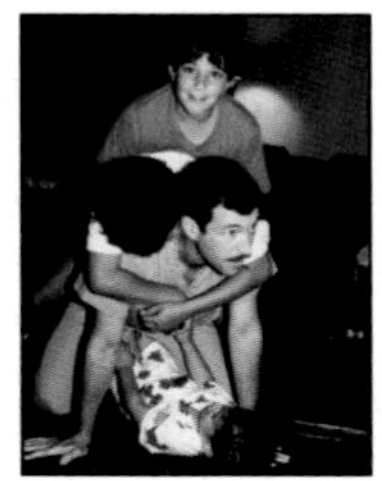

CHAPTER 11

Lighten Up!

It has been said that laughter is the best medicine. I never learned this in medical school, and it may not meet the definition of a drug, yet I am convinced that every human being should seek happiness, and as a temporary fix, there is nothing quite like laughter.

There is something very special about a warm smile that is transformed by laughter. While everybody's laugh is a bit different, ranging from a few snorts to a belly roar, what is shared in common is happiness.

A couple of rules are necessary to maximize the frequency and genuineness of laughter. First, we need to take ourselves less seriously. It is okay to spill food on our tie and laugh about it. While it is not usually appropriate to laugh at others, it is always good to laugh at one's self. In fact, it is absolutely healthy to do so. Second, while funny things happen to everybody, we need to intentionally look for humor in life because we only find what we are looking for (Figures 11-1 through 11-9).

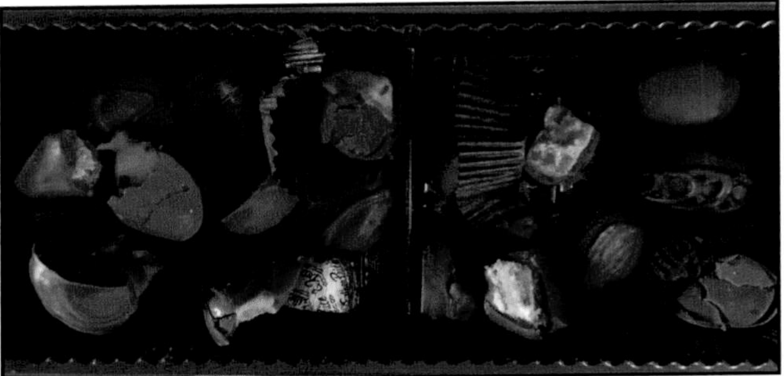

Figure 11-1. Special box of expensive chocolates for guests.

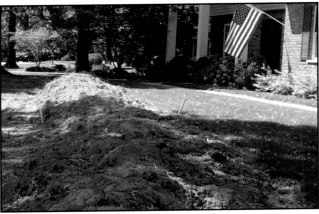

Figure 11-2. They have a real mole problem!

Several additional suggestions include having access to a few movies that are guaranteed to make you laugh. For example, there is something about the scene in *My Cousin Vinny* where the slick New York attorney has to show up in court wearing a rented costume in front of the austere judge that is guaranteed to hit my funny bone.

Figure 11-3. Time to change the outhouse!

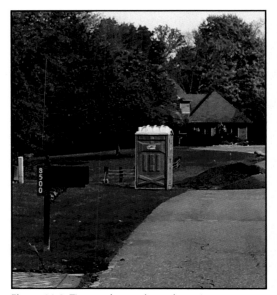

Figure 11-4. Are you really serious about finding your lucky golf ball?

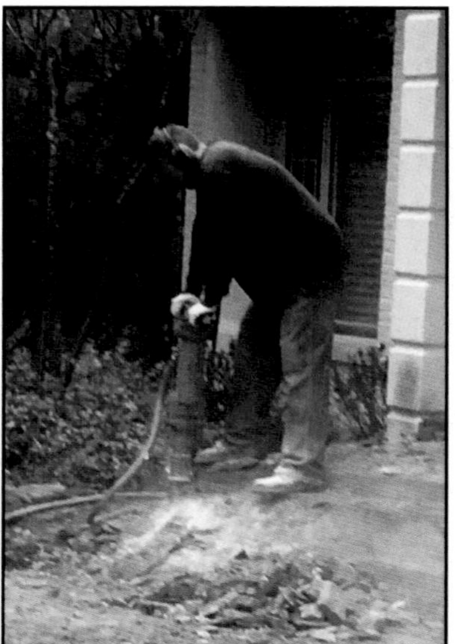

Figure 11-5. Future cataract surgeon.

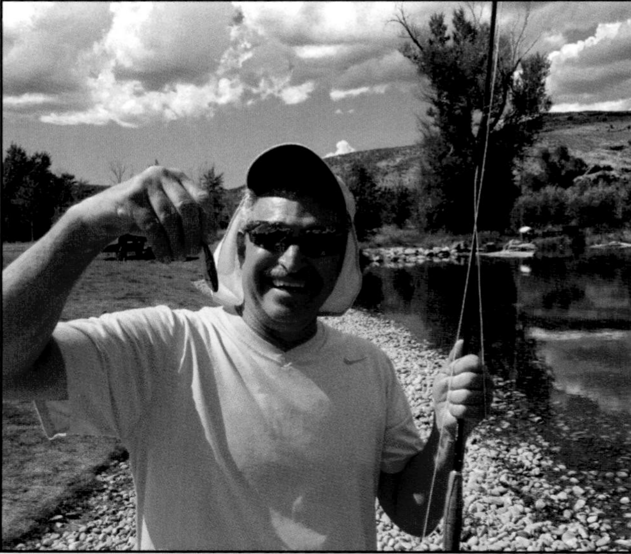

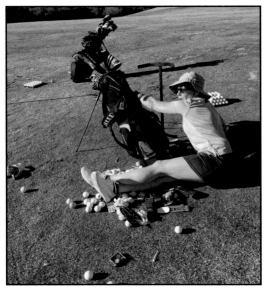

Figure 11-6. Fishing all day for this? !*!&?!%#!

My father taught me to write down a joke if it was particularly funny and then to share it with others. Dr. Spencer Thornton, a dear friend in Nashville, Tennessee, just sent me a story about a golfer, accompanied by his wife, who rushed into a dentist's office looking repeatedly at his watch. He told the dentist that an acute toothache was jeopardizing his 10:00 am tee time. The dentist explained that a tooth that had suddenly become painful might need to be pulled and might require some local anesthesia. The husband replied that there was no need for anesthesia because there was no time for anesthesia, and if necessary, to just go ahead and pull the tooth.

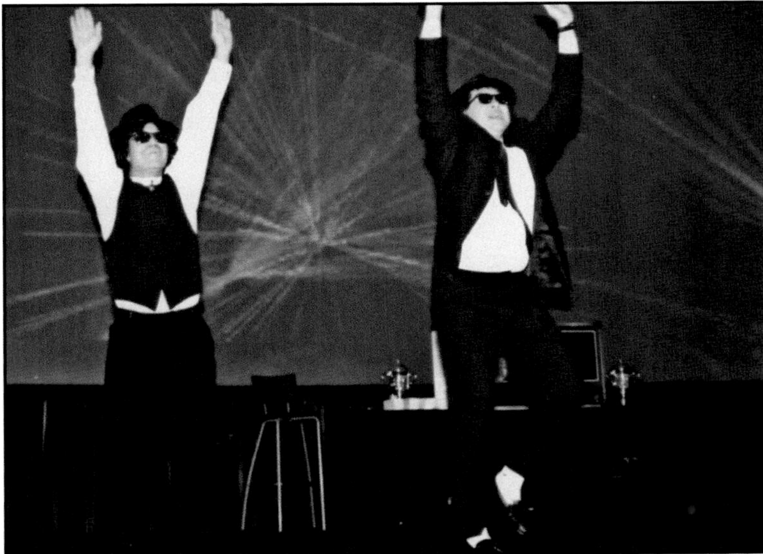

Figure 11-7. Internationally renowned cataract surgeon Dr. David Chang insisted that I accompany him on stage in a Blues Brothers routine. A career of earning a reputation as a serious educator was sacrificed in an instant for my good friend from California.

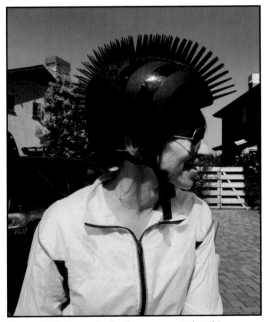

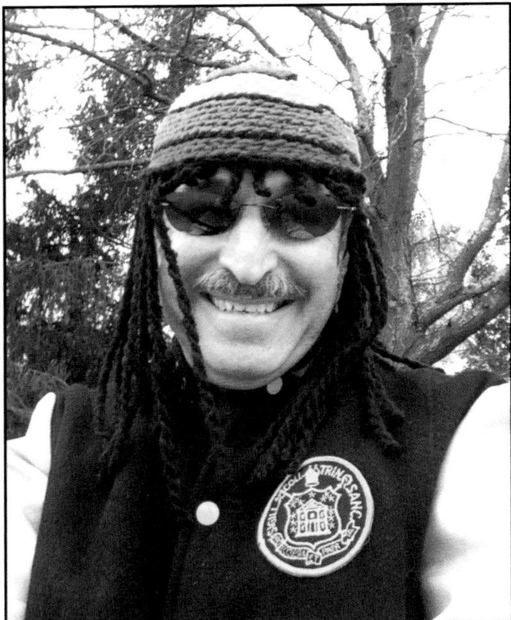

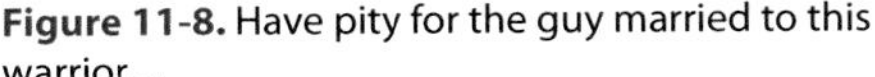

Figure 11-8. Have pity for the guy married to this warrior...

Figure 11-9. ...oh, that would be me!

The dentist asked the husband which tooth was the problem, and the husband replied, "Honey, open your mouth and show him!"

I love to laugh, and I enjoy being around people who love to laugh. I bought a joke book to be able to tell my young grandchildren something that will make them laugh: Why did the orange stop halfway up the stairs? Because it ran out of juice! Why did the banana stay home from school? Because it wasn't peeling well!

In this book written about the anatomy of Achievement, it is important to be serious about focusing on the goals that you set for yourself in order to achieve. Yet, this book is also about Balance, and we cannot be serious or take ourselves too seriously all of the time. So, kick back and laugh often…it is good for the soul!

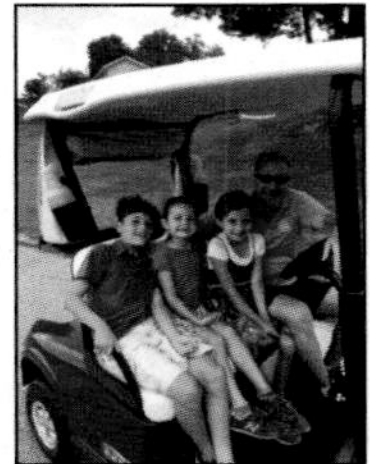

CHAPTER 12

The Hands of a Surgeon

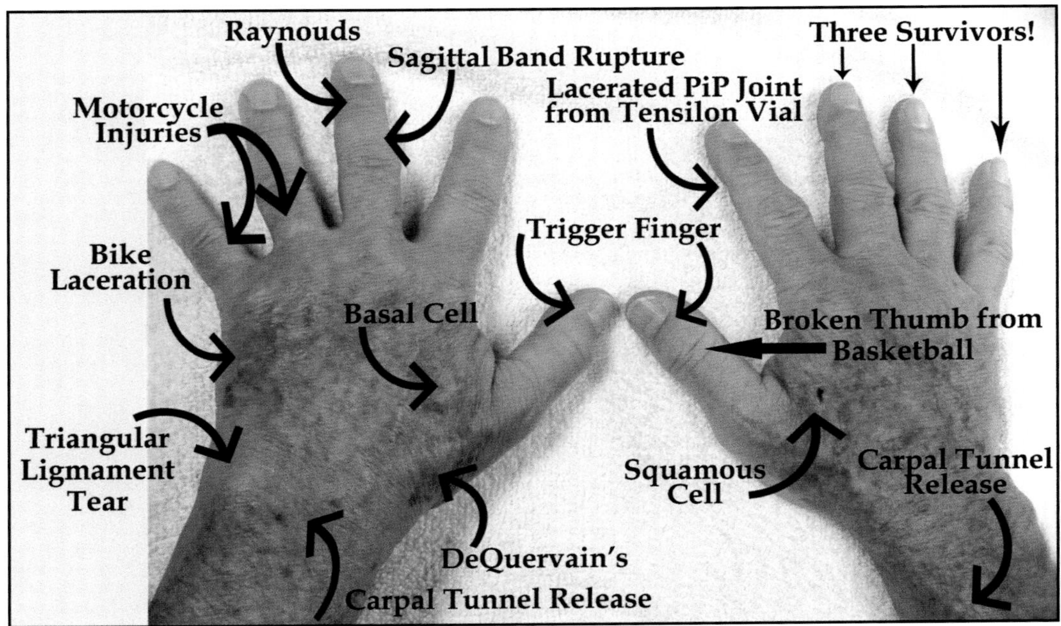

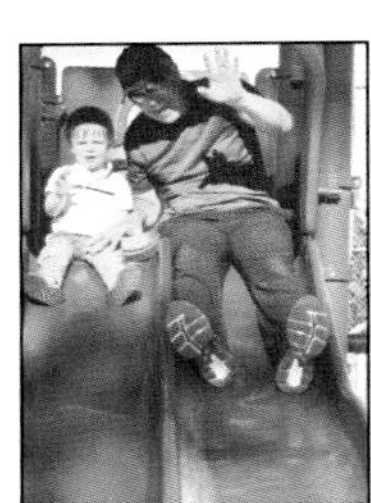

CHAPTER 13

Competition

There are few joys in life that exceed the thrill of competition. Throughout our childhoods and our adult careers, competition is ubiquitous, so it is advantageous to learn how to flourish as a competitor at an early age. Regardless of whether we are competing on the sports field, in the business world, or against ourselves on the golf course, feeling comfortable as a competitor is essential to becoming an achiever.

There are authorities who believe that competitive pressure can be destructive, and they are correct. However, the individual who becomes incapacitated under pressure is not the surgeon who I want operating on me. The athlete who cannot perform when the score is tied as the clock winds down is unlikely to experience the thrill of a last-minute victory. If we are honest and willing to admit that competition is as much a part of the American way of life as baseball and apple pie, society must ask how to best prepare our youth for a lifetime of healthy competition. Actually, if we are just willing to acknowledge the importance of competition, then we are already taking a gigantic step toward gaining a competitive edge.

There is a basic desire deep down within each of us to perform well and to succeed. I believe that this desire is intrinsic and can be observed when a youngster is tossing a ball into the air as he or she plays an imaginary game of baseball: "...and the ball is smashed deep toward the left field fence...going back...back...he leaps and makes a great catch, winning the game!" Our imaginations are constantly engaged in competitive exercises. The sooner children are exposed to the concept of competition, the easier it becomes to acquire a level of comfort when competing. This is why I have tried to expose each of my children and those whom I have coached to as many competitive situations as possible (see Figure 16-10). It is important that we talk about what it takes to become a winner and why success is never easy. The clear message is that becoming a consistent winner is only possible through desire, hard work, and mental toughness.

It has been interesting to observe how prevalent competition is among professionals. I quickly observed that there is a real territorialism that causes human beings to be protective of their turf and to behave aggressively toward any challenger. In the early years of my career, my novel approach to surgical techniques was encouraged by few and disparaged by many. Sometimes, human nature is not pretty, and we climb the ladder of success by kissing the feet on the rung above us while kicking the head on the rung below us. If one is an achiever, the kicks seem to come from everywhere. Once this behavior is understood, we can learn to conduct our life competing with self-control and dignity. We can compete fiercely and tenaciously while, at the same time, treating our competitors with respect. If we win, we exemplify good sportsmanship.

Osher RH. *The Real ABCs: A Surgeon's Analysis and a Father's Legacy, Second Edition* (pp 53-56).

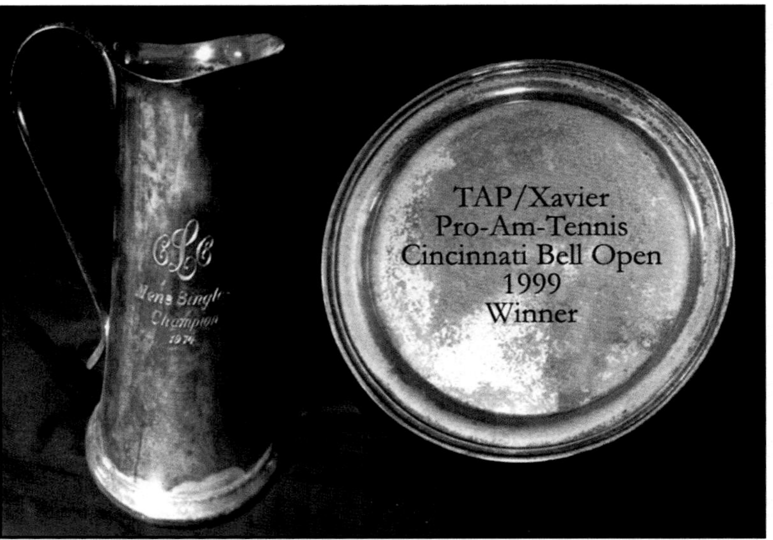

Figure 13-1. Tennis Club champion.

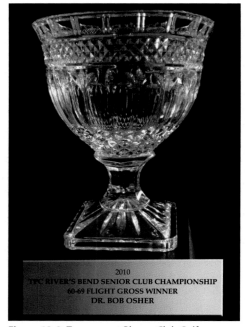

Figure 13-2. Tournament Players Club Golf championship.

If we are on the short end of the stick, we are able to accept defeat graciously, congratulating our adversary before analyzing the outcome and planning our course for improvement. My high school best friend, an attorney named Bob Brant, was never the most gifted athlete, but he always seemed to win because of his competitive toughness. Equally impressive was the fact that he was a real gentleman and one of the nicest guys in the world as he was dismantling his opponent.

I loved to compete as a youngster and even more as an adult. When my aging body started to resist my demands and expectations, I found other ways to continue to compete. When I could no longer run a respectable 10K, play a serious game of hoops, or play competitive tennis at a high level (Figure 13-1), I turned to biking, swimming, and kayaking and competed against the clock. I discovered the game of golf and competed against the course. My golfing buddies have even accused me of "sandbagging" my handicap (between 5 and 6) because I consistently shoot below it when the pressure is on. So, I prefer to compete using "gross" scores rather than a handicap, which is how I was able to win my age group in the senior championships at two different golf clubs (Figures 13-2 and 13-3). The reader is probably thinking that there was nobody else in my age group—not true!

Early on, I began coaching multiple sports, and the youngsters on 70 teams over 3 decades have witnessed my competitive spirit and sportsmanship (Figures 13-4 and 13-5). I also entered international surgery competitions (Film Festivals), and my videos were critiqued and graded against the finest surgeons on the planet. After more than 40 top awards, I am still just as excited every time the nine international judges bring out the envelopes and announce the winner (Figures 13-6 and 13-7). I even like to compete when the competition is just for fun (Figure 13-8).

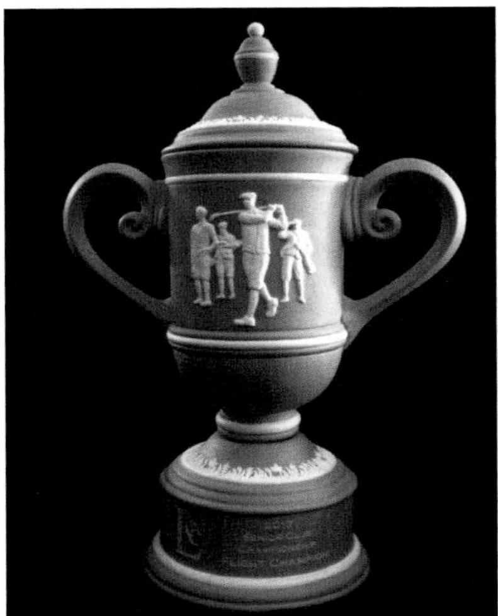

Figure 13-3. Losantiville Golf Champion Ages 60 to 69.

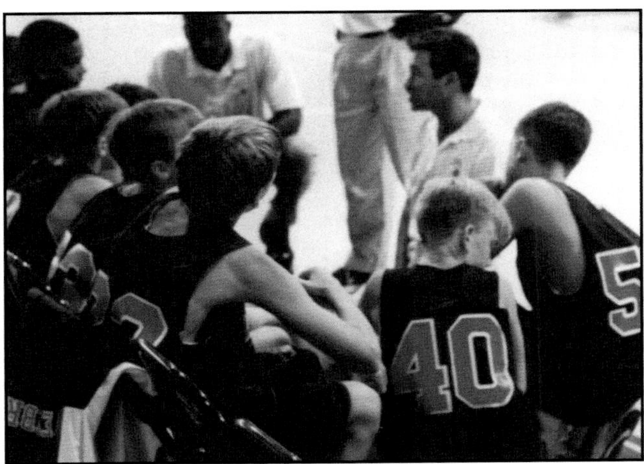

Figure 13-4. Coaching at the Amateur Athletic Union National Championships at Disney World.

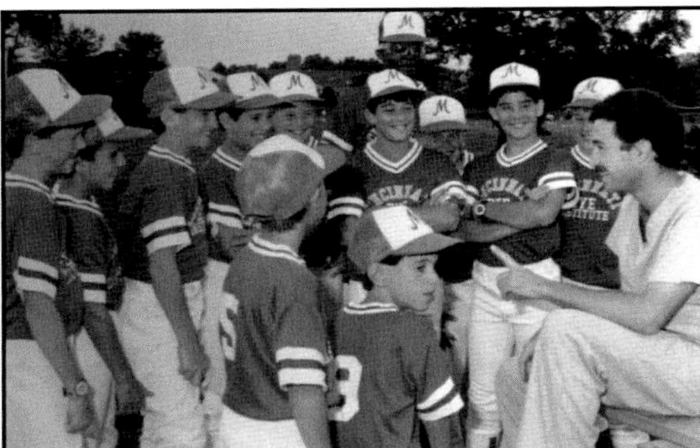

Figure 13-5. Rushing from the OR to the baseball field or basketball court for decades.

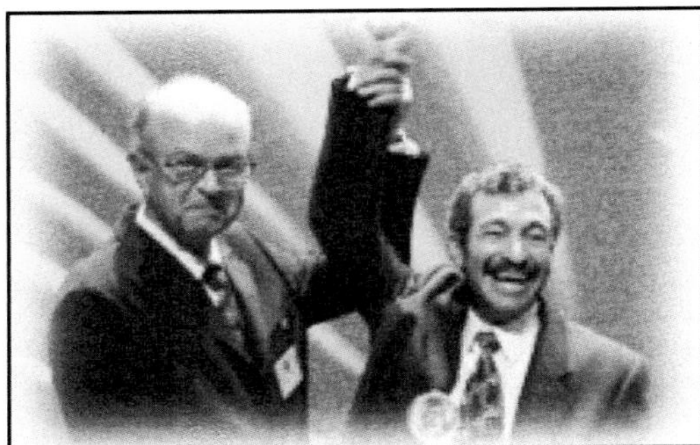

Figure 13-6. Winning the Film Festival in Europe.

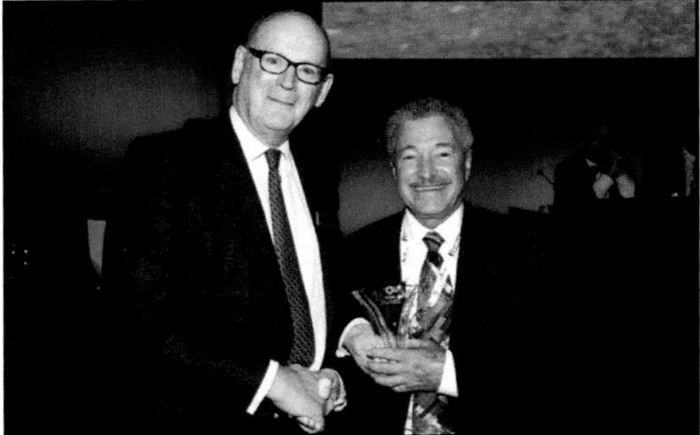

Figure 13-7. More subdued, but just as excited 30 years later!

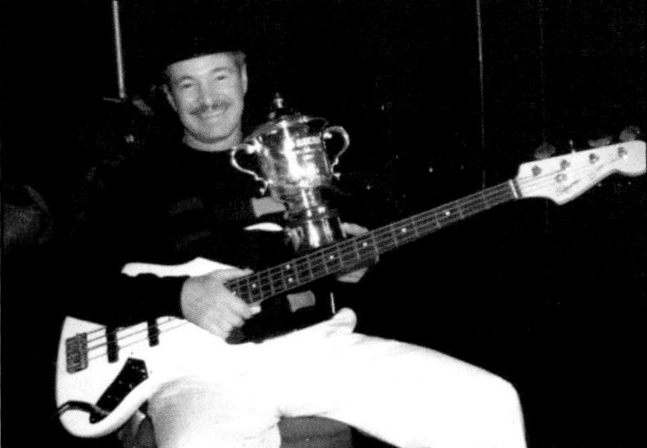

Figure 13-8. The American Cataract Society used to sponsor the Challenge Cup where multiple teams would present education in an entertaining fashion. Despite the fact that we were far from the Beatles and the judges were tone deaf, victory was ever so sweet.

Competition is the American way of life, and in order to reach our Achievement potential, we should be prepared to compete regardless of the outcome while dealing comfortably with and respectfully toward our competitors.

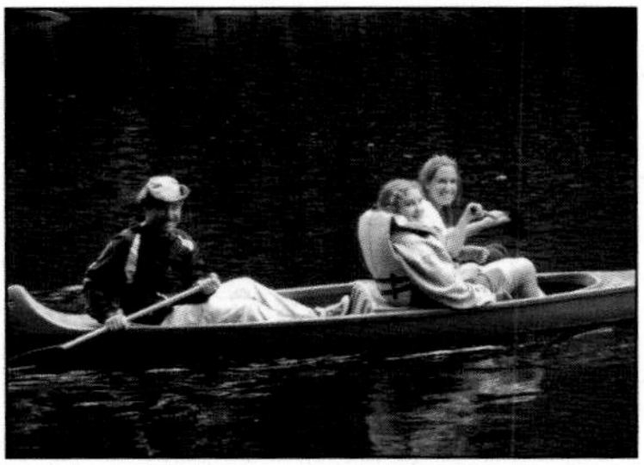

CHAPTER 14

Teaching

The Privilege of Giving Back

How ironic is it that, in our great society, professional athletes are paid millions of dollars each year while our teachers, the gatekeepers of our minds, have minimal economic value by comparison? Today, almost nothing, except professional athletics and CEO jobs in Silicon Valley, can be accomplished without higher education, and I would bet that each of our lives has been influenced by a handful of gifted and enthusiastic teachers.

After completing my training in ophthalmology and 3 additional fellowship years to acquire extra ophthalmic expertise, I made a commitment that I would devote one-quarter of my time to teaching. I have always had enormous respect for the outstanding teachers who have shaped my life and I, in turn, wanted to give back by positively shaping the lives of others.

In my profession, there are several ways to teach. Lecturing at the local medical school is one option. Another proven method is to give presentations at scientific meetings. There is also an opportunity to offer a clinical fellowship or preceptorship to medical students, residents, and postgraduate physicians. For those who are very ambitious, authoring a textbook is an endless labor of love. In the specialty of cataract surgery, another teaching opportunity involves entering the international Film Festivals. In these competitions, a surgeon produces a video unveiling a new technology, demonstrating the management of challenging case, or showcasing some innovative clinical technique. Perhaps the most prestigious teaching opportunity is an invitation to speak to an eye society or to address a national/international congress. All of these activities require time and effort, not to mention that an invitation is required to lecture. Moreover, traveling today has drawbacks such as delayed or missed flights, sleeping in noisy hotels, and getting hosed by local taxi drivers. Although teaching has little or no associated financial reward, many of the best things in life do not have a monetary benefit. As mentioned earlier, one should never confuse net worth with self-worth.

In the early 1980s, I designed an intraocular lens for cataract surgery that was produced by a handful of companies including Johnson & Johnson, Intermedics Inc, and 3M. To my surprise, the lens became one of the most popular lenses used in the United States, which led to a number of lecture invitations. I found that it was very satisfying to show my colleagues how to use the lens, and my initial anxiety for public speaking seemed to disappear. At about the same time, I was traveling every few weeks to visit different well-known cataract surgeons who were often located a long way from Cincinnati, Ohio. I did not relish spending a lot of money to take a 1-day trip requiring a lengthy plane ride, but it was the only way to be certain that I was providing the most contemporary techniques to my patients. Then, I had a wonderful idea: why not invite each of these leading surgeons to record their technique, which I could then edit

Osher RH. *The Real ABCs: A Surgeon's Analysis and a Father's Legacy, Second Edition* (pp 57-63).

Figure 14-1. Learning to edit the *Audiovisual Journal of Cataract & Implant Surgery.*

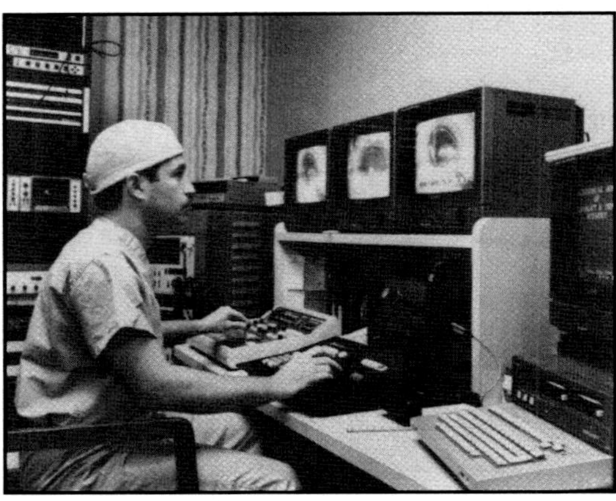

JANUARY 15, 1985 5

Video cataract journal makes 1985 debut

CINCINNATI—*The Audiovisual Journal of Cataract & Implant Surgery,* a quarterly videocassette featuring sections on phacoemulsification, planned and automated extracapsular extraction techniques, complication management, and literature review and viewpoints, should be available to cataract surgeons early this year, said Robert H. Osher, MD, in an interview with OCULAR SURGERY NEWS.

"After speaking with many surgeons, I became convinced that the best way to improve surgical skills was not by hearing or reading about them, but by watching and scrutinizing another surgeon's operating technique," explained Dr. Osher, who will serve as the journal's editor. "It became apparent that surgeons can not only learn better techniques, but that the new media, videotape, can let them view complications and the management of those complications firsthand.

"This project brings the leading surgeons in the cataract field into your living room," he added, "where you can glean their tricks and pearls at your convenience. And the response so far has been marvelous."

Guest physicians appearing in the first issue of the videocassette journal include Dr. Osher, Antonio Mendez, MD, Robert C. Drews, MD, Richard P. Kratz, MD, David J. McIntyre, MD, Thomas R. Mazzocco, MD, and Walter J. Stark, MD.

The yearly subscription rate will be $200, which includes four one-hour programs on either VHS, Beta, or ¾" videocassette. The journal is supported in part by educational grants from Iolab, Pharmacia, 3M, American Medical Optics, Alcon, and CooperVision. For subscription information, contact: Cincinnati Eye Institute, 10496 Montgomery Road, Cincinnati, Ohio 45242. ■

Figure 14-2. Announcing the debut of the first video journal in medicine.

into a video program reaching colleagues in the United States and abroad (Figure 14-1)? This was the birth of the *Audiovisual Journal of Cataract & Implant Surgery*, the first video journal in medicine (Figure 14-2). I had stumbled onto a unique method of continuing surgical education that would allow the viewer to sit comfortably in his or her living room, munching on a favorite snack, while learning from master surgeons around the world. Within several years, the *Audiovisual Journal* was being viewed by large audiences in more than 150 countries, and I was busy compiling new techniques, challenging cases, examples of complications, and new technologies for an hour-long program every 3 months. The educational impact of the *Audiovisual Journal* was unparalleled, and, after a name change to the *Video Journal of Cataract & Refractive Surgery*, it is now a free member benefit of almost every cataract society in the world.

From my first day in private practice, I decided to record all of my operations on video. This obsessive behavior resulted in a remarkable teaching collection. At the national and international meetings in the early 1980s, I would present unusual situations, especially complications that no other surgeon dared to show. In fact, virtually every speaker showed a near flawless procedure in contrast to my presentations, which demonstrated the management of a challenging problem or an unexpected complication. The interest was so high that I was able to introduce a new teaching format, "The Video Symposium," featuring my toughest cases. Suddenly, my presentations were in great demand, and I was receiving a steady stream of invitations from ophthalmology societies around the United States. The *Video Journal* was also developing quite an international following, and speaking invitations began to pour in from cataract societies in Europe, Asia, Japan, Australia, and South America (Figure 14-3). Faced with the dilemma of wanting to teach but not wanting to miss work (nor did I wish to be away from my family), I

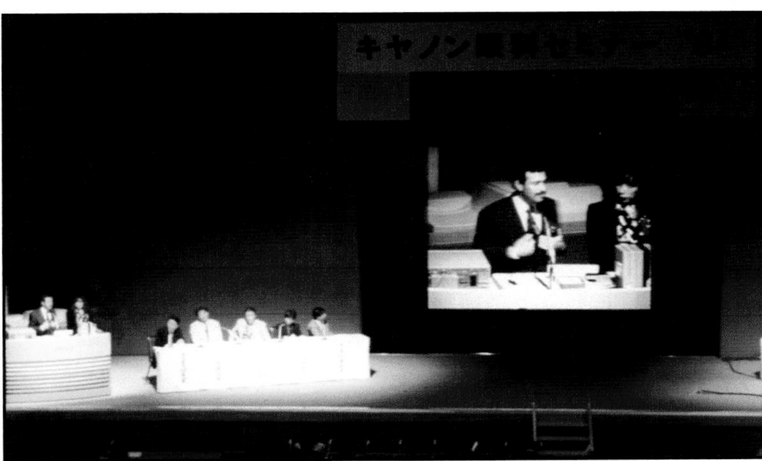

Figure 14-3. Guest Speaker at the Japanese Cataract Congress.

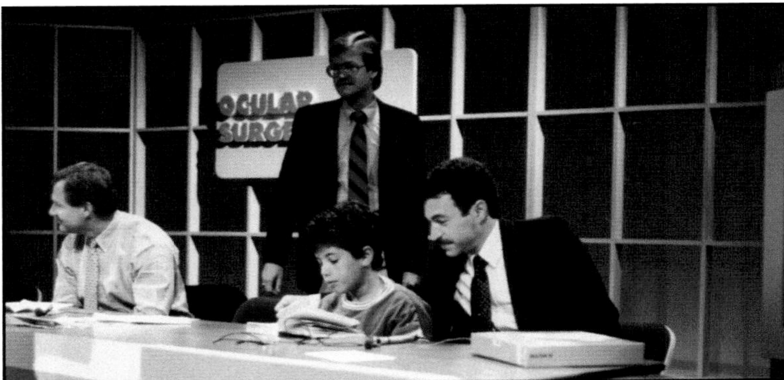

Figure 14-4. Enjoying my son's company between lectures. He is now a retinal surgeon and one of my associates.

would fly to international destinations, dash to the lecture site, present several hours of videos, and then head back to the airport! By 1990, I was logging approximately 100,000 miles each year in a plane. If the lecture site was closer to home, I often would take one of my youngsters with me as a way of combining the pleasure of teaching with enjoyable quality time with one of my kids (Figure 14-4).

This was my "modus operandi" for years until my body began to object to this grueling style of international travel, so I changed my approach. Instead, I would arrive, teach, and then take 1 or 2 extra days to explore the Amazon, adventure though the crocodile-infested swampland of northern Australia (Figure 14-5), balloon over the Alps, or dive amongst the sharks off the coast of Bali. Still, the primary purpose of these excursions was always to educate other eye surgeons.

My love for teaching, my willingness to travel, and my zeal for new technology and techniques led to invitations to teach in fascinating places (Figure 14-6). My courses were usually packed with standing room only (Figure 14-7), probably because I was never reluctant to show my most difficult cases. I suspect that audiences found it enjoyable to observe another surgeon "sweating bullets" while struggling to get out of trouble, which made for highly effective teaching. Today, I am truly humbled to have the unique opportunity to present my own prime-time symposium at the three major meetings: the American Academy of Ophthalmology, the American Society of Cataract and Refractive Surgery, and the European Society of Cataract and Refractive Surgeons. Just last week in Paris, I was caught by surprise as the President of the European Society of Cataract & Refractive Surgeons presented me with a first-time special award for teaching (Figure 14-8).

Figure 14-5. Exploring the Australian wilderness by helicopter.

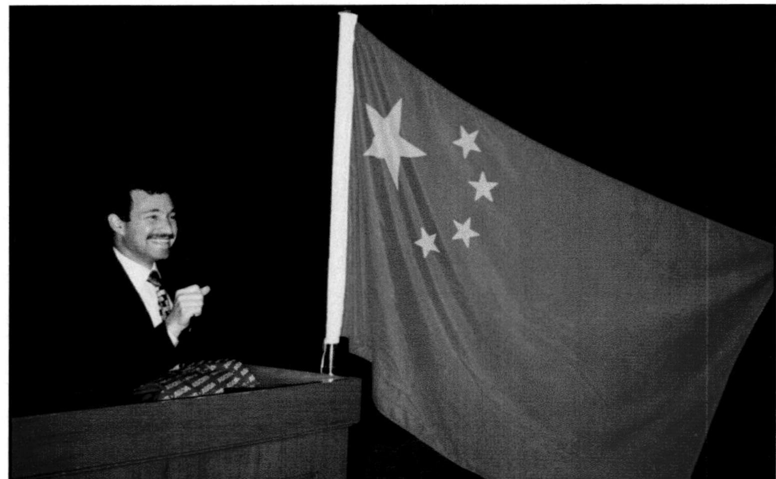

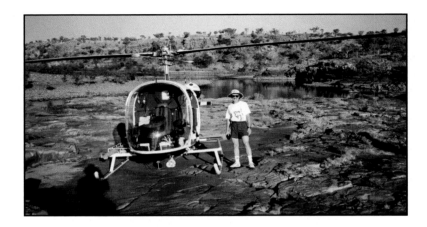

Figure 14-6. The Chinese interpreter must have inspired the movie *Lost in Translation*.

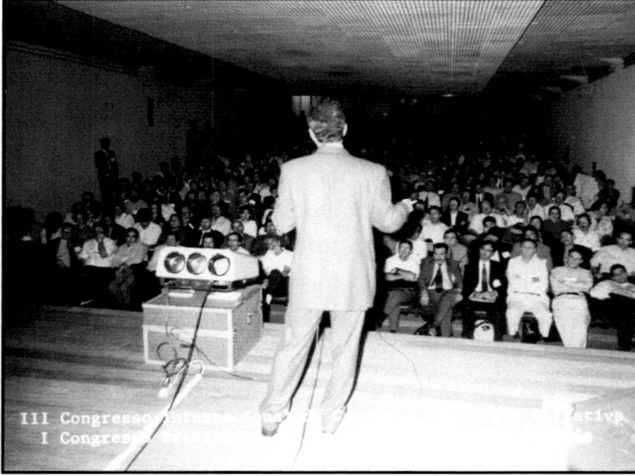

Figure 14-7. Standing room audience in Brazil.

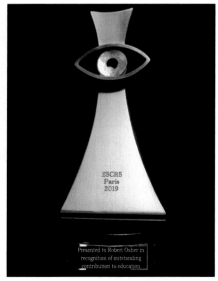

Figure 14-8. Unexpected award for decades of educating colleagues at the Annual Meeting of the European Society of Cataract and Refractive Surgeons.

Figure 14-9. Writing textbooks—a necessary evil.

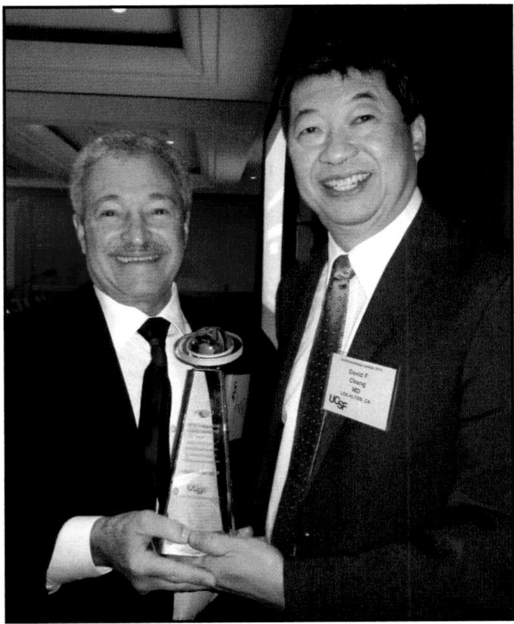

Figure 14-10. A great privilege to deliver the Inaugural Chang Lecture at University of California, San Francisco, honoring my dear friend and internationally renowned cataract surgeon, David Chang, MD.

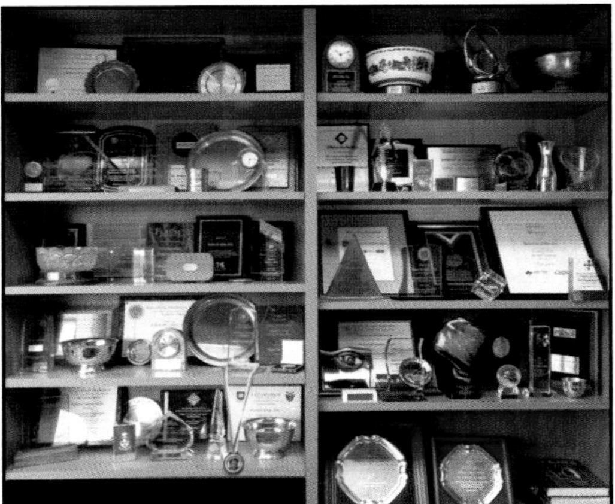

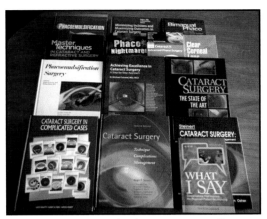

Figure 14-11. Memorabilia from named lectures.

Publishing is another essential way to effectively teach. I have spent an enormous number of hours writing, revising, proofing, and correcting manuscripts, articles, chapters, and even textbooks (Figure 14-9). It is never easy to publish, nor is it especially enjoyable. Yet, journals are the scientific foundation for communication among cataract surgeons, and in some years, I have published as many as 12 peer-reviewed articles while serving on countless editorial boards. I view this work as a necessary evil. Dr. Bob Kersten, one of America's most talented oculoplastic surgeons, compares publishing a chapter in a textbook to reaching first base by getting hit by the pitch!

Named lectures constitute a very special invitation because the lecture represents a tribute to a person who is making or has made a major medical contribution prior to his or her death. The named lecture usually is the highlight of a meeting, and there is often a small award or plaque that the speaker receives to commemorate the occasion (Figure 14-10). It has been my privilege to deliver more than 50 named lectures, which allow me to both teach and honor the memory of a colleague (Figure 14-11).

Mentoring young surgeons provides another option for teaching. For years, I offered a postgraduate fellowship in cataract surgery. This extra training for a surgeon about to begin his or her practice is extremely helpful in polishing skills and gaining confidence after completing the required training to become an ophthalmologist. I have enjoyed training many young surgeons,

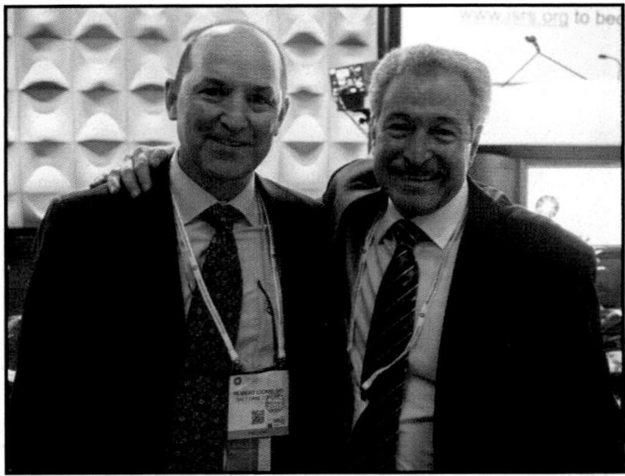

Figure 14-12. Dr. Robert Cionni, a former Fellow, received the Kelman Award from the American Academy of Ophthalmology.

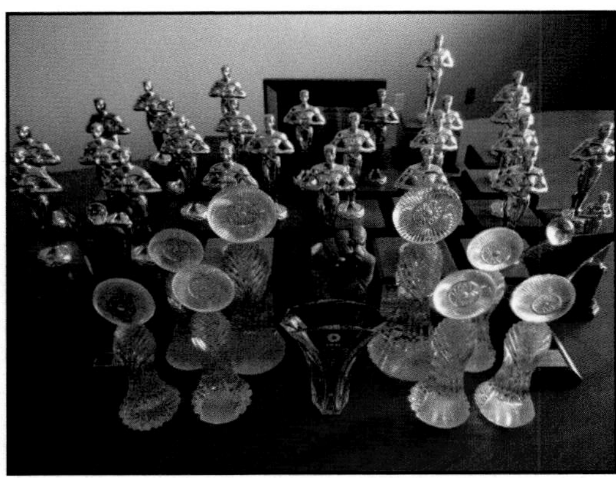

Figure 14-13. Does the hardware reflect the hard work?

but none more accomplished than Dr. Robert Cionni, who ascended to the Presidency of the American Society of Cataract and Refractive Surgery. His innovative contributions in managing challenging cases brought both international recognition and prestigious awards to this outstanding surgeon (Figure 14-12).

In my opinion, the ultimate teaching activity in ophthalmology is the international cataract surgery video competition, otherwise known as the Film Festival in America and the Video Competition in Europe. The surgeon has 1 year to conceptualize an educational goal, perform the required surgeries, write the script, edit and narrate the video, and then add music and special effects. The judging panel consists of nine international surgeons who spend several days in isolation scrutinizing hundreds of entries for educational content and artistic merit. The Film Festival ceremony is a black-tie event with the same electricity as the Academy Awards, including the champagne, the orchestra, and a boisterous audience consisting of several thousand physicians and members of the industry. The winners are awarded gold statues quite similar to the Oscars. I have received three Grand Prizes in the American, European, and Asian competitions in addition to more than 40 first or second place awards (Figure 14-13). Although the organizing committee has invited me to retire and join the judging panel, I just cannot walk away from the thrill of the competition!

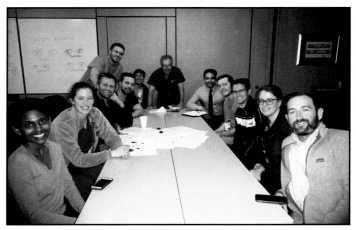

Figure 14-14. These bright residents keep me on my toes!

Even though I have been teaching for about 40 years, I still look forward to every major meeting as well as my quaint evening dinner conferences with the ophthalmology residents at the University of Cincinnati (Figure 14-14). I also still enjoy giving Grand Rounds, although getting up at 6:00 am is no longer pleasant. The plaque that I received from the residents as "Teacher of the Year" remains one of my career favorites (Figure 14-15).

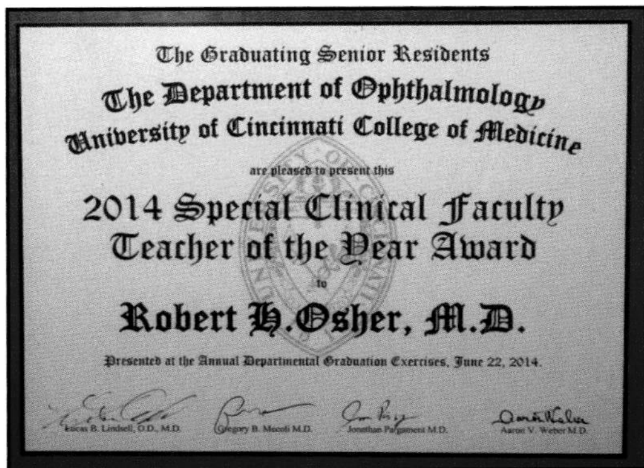

Figure 14-15. Prized Teacher of the Year Award.

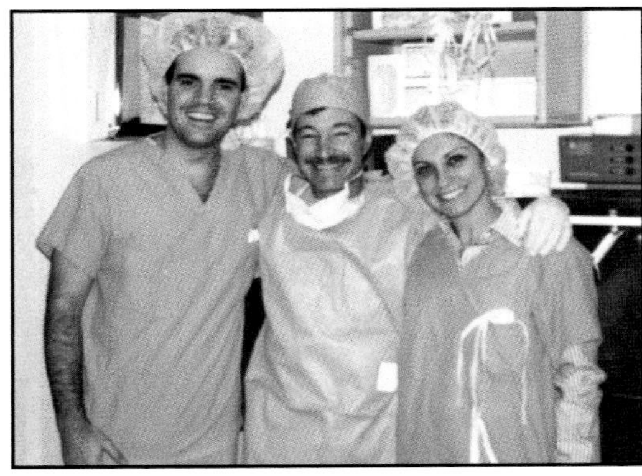

Figure 14-16. Outstanding Fellows, Fred and Dani Marques from Brazil make teaching a joy!

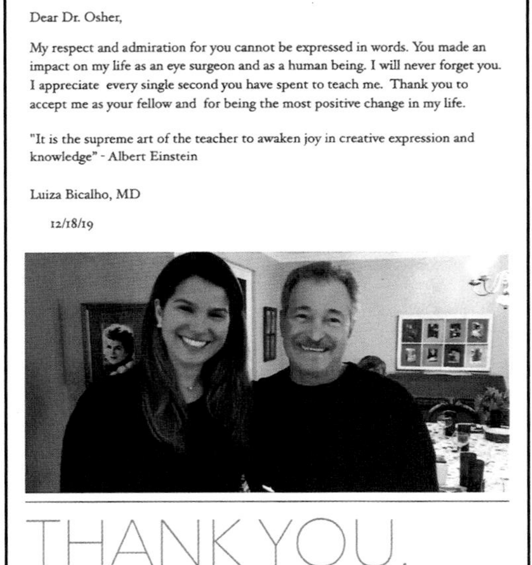

Dear Dr. Osher,

My respect and admiration for you cannot be expressed in words. You made an impact on my life as an eye surgeon and as a human being. I will never forget you. I appreciate every single second you have spent to teach me. Thank you to accept me as your fellow and for being the most positive change in my life.

"It is the supreme art of the teacher to awaken joy in creative expression and knowledge" - Albert Einstein

Luiza Bicalho, MD

12/18/19

THANK YOU.

Figure 14-17. It's been a privilege to teach visiting surgeons for four decades.

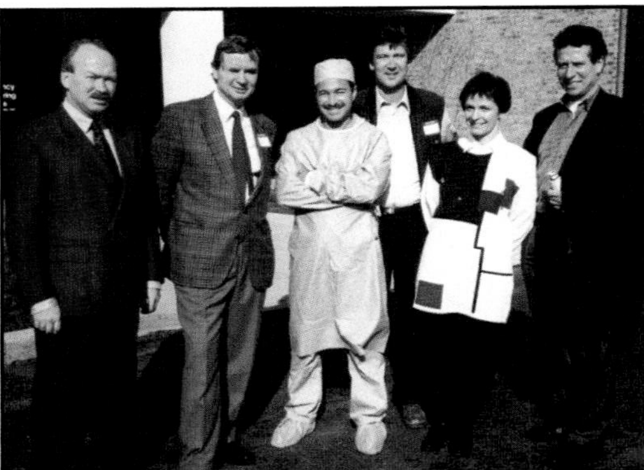

Figure 14-18. Hosting a delegation of cataract surgeons from Germany.

The key to becoming a teacher is to decide to do it early in a career and then to work diligently toward this goal. While the awards and recognition are nice, there is a distinct sense of accomplishment derived from training residents/fellows (Figure 14-16), teaching a group of young surgeons the "tricks of the trade," hosting a visiting surgeon (Figure 14-17), or hosting an international ophthalmic delegation (Figure 14-18). Granted, there may be little financial compensation for the endless number of hours writing, editing, and traveling to lecture, but teaching is one of the true privileges in medicine. There is great satisfaction in both sharing knowledge and in influencing the careers of other surgeons.

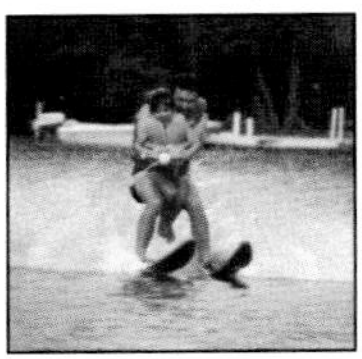

CHAPTER 15

What Goes Around... Comes Around

You really cannot make up stories like this one. Let's go back about 30 years when a very young and enthusiastic cataract surgeon received an invitation to chair the morning session of a very popular meeting in Hawaii called the *Royal Hawaiian Eye Meeting* (RHEM). The meeting was scheduled in January every year, the venue rotating from island to island. A half day Sunday through the following Friday was spent covering the different subspecialties, leaving the remainder of time for attendees to enjoy amazing outdoor activities. Two mornings were devoted to cataract surgery, and I was given the opportunity to chair one of them. I took my responsibility very seriously and was always overly prepared, which resulted in high evaluations leading to 15 years of encore performances.

Then, I was approached by another group that was interested in breaking away from the original RHEM. Two very influential surgeons from Boston, Massachusetts said that they were interested in founding a more scientific meeting, and they made an offer that I could not refuse. They offered to give me more speaking time and were willing to cover my rather hefty expenses, including a first-class ticket as well as the pricey hotel. They also appealed to my academic background, and one of the surgeons, Roger Steinert, MD, was a very close friend. Therefore, I chose to join the mutiny and follow them to another island, where they scheduled their meeting at virtually the same time as the RHEM. For the next 5 years or so, it was a very good decision, and I had no regrets as this new meeting became very popular.

However, two large ophthalmic meetings in Hawaii during January created a real conundrum for the industry supporting these meetings with their exhibit fees and promotional meals. Protests grew louder until a large publishing company, The Wyanoke Group, purchased the two meetings and consolidated the faculty into one, much to the delight of the industry. I continued to chair a portion of the meeting that dealt with complication management during cataract surgery and another session that The Wyanoke Group had requested dealing with new technology. The former topic was my strength, but I agreed to also organize the latter because of the explosion of new technology that had made the field of cataract surgery so exciting year after year. Moreover, I had chaired a similar session at the Annual Meeting of the American Academy of Ophthalmology, which was very popular and attracted thousands of surgeons interested in learning about new technology. I was very careful to include all of the companies with new products, and I selected a balanced panel of surgeons who used the products from many different companies. In other words, I did my best to create an even playing field for both speakers and products. Now, the plot thickens.

Osher RH. *The Real ABCs: A Surgeon's Analysis and a Father's Legacy, Second Edition* (pp 65-68).

About 10 years ago, I received a note in the mail sent from Vindico Medical Education, the educational division of The Wyanoke Group, which informed me that I was being suspended for 1 year. The reason: I had violated the new Continuing Medical Education (CME) guidelines. The note went on to explain that I was no longer allowed to use product names, a violation that required a mandatory suspension according to their zero-tolerance protocol. I wrote back that the title of my symposium was, "New Products in Cataract Surgery" and how was I possibly supposed to deliver this impartial, unbiased symposium without mentioning product names? Perhaps I was supposed to pantomime the discussion! Moreover, I reminded the educational committee that THEY had assigned this topic to me. It was so ridiculous because I had just given a similar presentation to a standing-room crowd at the American Academy of Ophthalmology, and there were no objections from the most conservative, law-abiding organization on the planet.

There was no possibility that I was going to let this group of "education police," who had never given a single lecture, intimidate me into submission. Therefore, I refused their 1-year suspension and instead insisted that the penalty be a LIFETIME BAN! That is when I decided to start my own meeting.

I sought out a small group composed of some of the ultra-talented surgeons who were also respected educators. They were highly confident truth-seekers who shared my indignation and rebellious nature. Their credentials were above reproach, and they became the small but exceptional faculty of a new meeting entitled *Cataract Surgery: Telling It Like It Is!* Our singular goal was to provide the highest-quality education for cataract surgeons who believed in unrestricted, free speech and wanted to deliver the best possible care to their patients, even if it meant not receiving CME credit for their attendance. That's right, this was the first "educational" meeting with absolutely no CME. The naysayers predicted that the meeting would fail miserably because academic credit was not being given. Fortunately, as I learned from one of my favorite and most respected mentors, J. Lawton Smith, MD, "The truth is not defined by the majority opinion!"

The meeting started with a handful of exhibitors and a very small number of cataract surgeons who attended the inaugural conference at the Ritz-Carlton Hotel in Sarasota, Florida. I am sure that we violated every CME rule by reviewing cutting-edge techniques and unapproved devices that were being used outside of the United States. I even smuggled a few products into the country to share with attendees. The format was innovative with spirited discussions between the faculty and audience, punctuated by frequent disagreement among our experts. The education was candid and aimed at making every attendee a more knowledgeable and confident surgeon. We started the 4-day marathon at 7:00 am and finished at 11:00 pm every evening. The symposia were video-based and the wet labs allowed hands-on practice with artificial eyes (Figure 15-1). The meals were provided by the companies whose products were discussed, not by their own reps, but rather by respected surgeons who had experience using the technology. The evening sessions were casual and lighthearted; I enjoyed bringing the late-night snacks and serving the beer and pretzels to the audience. Attendees could ask any faculty member questions about a difficult case from home. The agenda targeted surgeons with varying levels of experience, and we invited all young residents still in training who could attend far below cost (I made up the difference myself). At the end of the conference, I asked every surgeon to fill out an evaluation with suggestions and criticisms, which I read religiously and used to select the new faculty and topics for the following year.

Cataract Surgery: Telling It Like It Is! experienced unprecedented success with explosive growth, and soon the meeting was attracting 600 cataract surgeons and more than 100 exhibitors (Figure 15-2). We outgrew Sarasota after 5 years, then outgrew Naples 2 years later. Our 9th meeting, held on Amelia Island in Florida, sold out the entire Ritz-Carlton Hotel and three nearby hotels. The faculty swelled to about 50 experts, and the meeting management was taken over

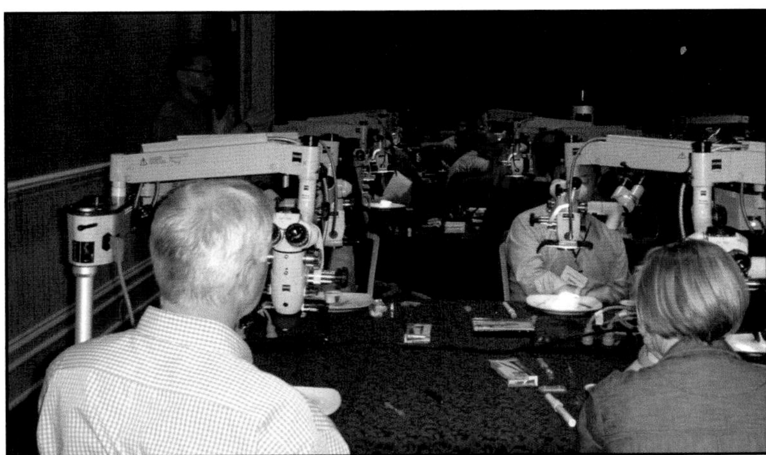

Figure 15-1. Wet labs offer hands-on practice.

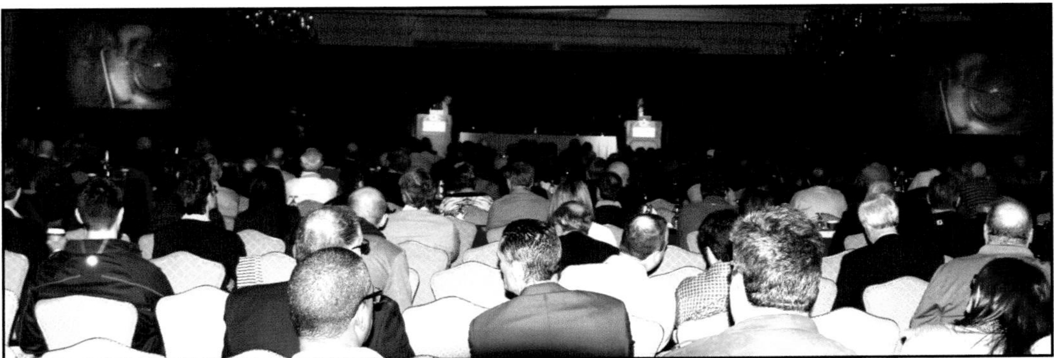

Figure 15-2. Audience is larger ever year.

by the American Academy of Ophthalmology. That was all very good, but behind the scenes, the meeting was taking a terrible toll on my personal life. I enjoyed the teaching, interacting with the faculty, and developing the agenda, but I hated the endless emails, negotiating with hotels, selecting menus, developing the marketing, organizing transportation, hiring security, creating the program with all of the advertisements, designing the signage, and working incessantly with the exhibitors. Every Christmas Eve, I was on my hands and knees laying out 113 exhibit spaces with masking tape! I could be in the middle of surgery when a telephone call would fracture the serenity of my operating room with an urgent message like, "The microscope is stuck in the freight elevator and you need to hire a forklift!" All of this was happening at the same time as I was juggling my busy practice, my lecture schedule, my research, my *Video Journal*, my fitness routine, building a relationship with Debbie, and my desire to spend time with five children and nine grandchildren. For the first time in my career, I did not have enough time to produce a competitive video for the American and European Film Festivals. Something just had to change.

I reached out to one of my very dear friends, Richard Lindstrom, MD, a remarkable ophthalmologist with very strong ties to the ophthalmic industry. I asked Dick if he knew of a respected company who might be interested in purchasing the meeting. Within 24 hours, he returned my call, indicating that he had found a buyer, but that I might want to sit down before he revealed the name...The Wyanoke Group! This was the very same company whose educational division had suspended me 10 years earlier and drove me to start my own meeting. I resisted the temptation to respond with a vociferous, "No #?!*!!* way!" In fact, I acquiesced to his suggestion to

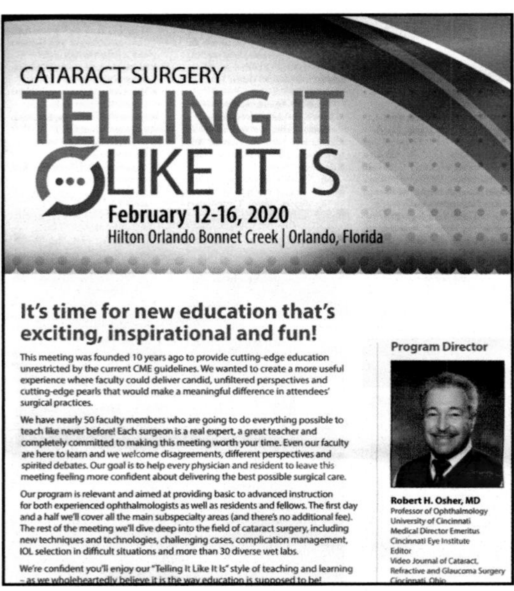

Figure 15-3. Marketing for Cataract Surgery: Telling It Like It Is!

set up a meeting with the owner, Peter Slack, which took place during the European Society of Cataract and Refractive Surgeons Congress in Lisbon, Portugal. The conversation was a bit awkward but cordial, and Peter came back with an offer that I quickly accepted. He insisted that I sign a 4-year contract to continue teaching and organizing the meeting, but everything else was The Wyanoke Group's responsibility. Hallelujah!

To my surprise, our first year working together exceeded all expectations. The Wyanoke Group team was professional, reliable, and honest, and our partnership turned out to be a genuine pleasure. The meeting was held at Disney World, an appropriate venue to celebrate getting my life back on track.

Since childhood, I have heard the expression, what goes around...comes around. I cannot think of a more perfect example, and I am so very optimistic about the meeting's future. As long as we attract the best faculty who can teach without restriction and have no fear of being gagged or shackled, both cataract surgeons and industry will find their way to Florida every winter to spend 1 week learning about new technology and improving surgical skills (Figure 15-3). However, unlike other tropical meetings, no one will return home with a tan!

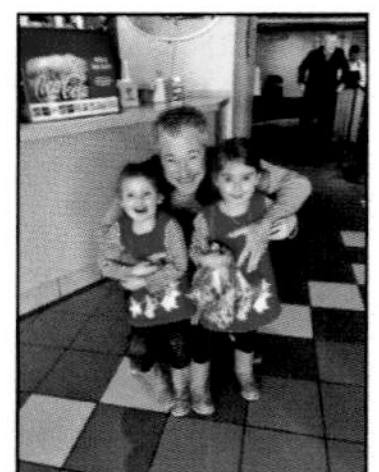

CHAPTER 16

Developing Our Next Generation

While I have placed a high value on teaching surgeons, I believe our lives are fullest when we can pass along something positive not only to colleagues through teaching, but also to the next generation. Besides, it is our duty in our role as the official caretakers of the future. There is a relatively brief window of opportunity for us to bequeath the values that will make our next generation a productive, secure, and happy bunch. We hold the powerful keys that will turn on and provide direction to our progeny.

When I was in college, I volunteered to teach boxing to youngsters in the Big Brothers organization in Hartford, Connecticut. I was fortunate to have boxed for Rolly Schwartz, a wonderful man who eventually became the United States Olympic boxing coach (Figure 16-1). I was never very talented, but that did not matter to Rolly. He loved the way I picked myself off the mat and returned to the battle, which no doubt contributed to my resiliency throughout life. I tried to convey this attitude when I was giving a boxing lesson, and I felt a great sense of satisfaction when working with kids.

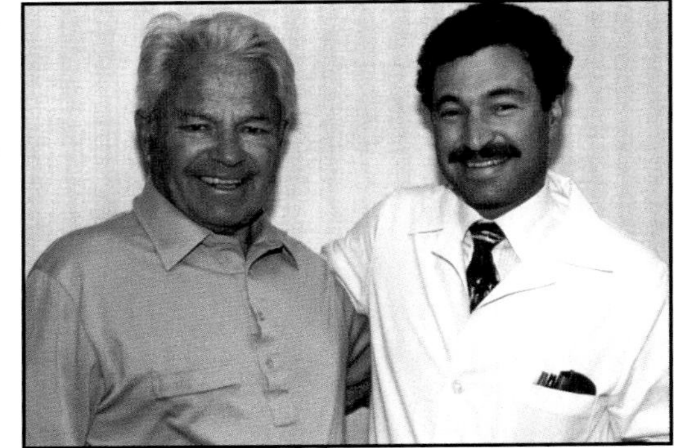

Figure 16-1. I learned boxing from Rolly Schwartz, USA Olympic coach.

When I arrived in medical school, I met Jeff Odel, another student who was also a talented magician from New York City. We struck up a friendship that has endured 4 decades, and Jeff taught me the art of card magic. Whenever the opportunity presented, I would stroll through the pediatric wards with a deck of cards for the sole purpose of bringing a smile to some child's face. Even when I fumbled the cards with my minimally skilled hands, the spontaneous laughter and the moment were very special. I was beginning to realize how much I enjoyed interacting with the next generation.

When I reflect about which people had a major influence on my life, the name Willard Stargell immediately comes to mind. Mr. Stargell was an African American athlete who had been a standout on the University of Cincinnati football team. He later joined the faculty of the large public high school that I attended and served as the head football coach. For some inexplicable reason, Mr. Stargell took an interest in me as I battled to make the basketball team. Even though my father stood over 6 feet tall, I had been betrayed by my pituitary gland, and my lack of growth hormone distinguished me as one of the shortest kids in the class. My outside shot

Osher RH. *The Real ABCs: A Surgeon's Analysis and a Father's Legacy, Second Edition* (pp 69-76).

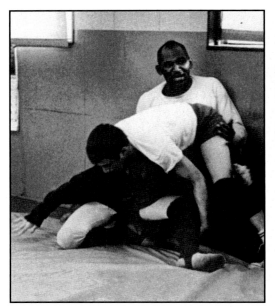

Figure 16-2. Willard Stargell helped me start the wrestling team.

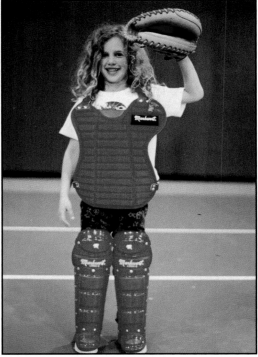

Figure 16-3. Jenny, my 5-year-old daughter, outplayed the boys.

was among the best in town, but I was neither quick nor able to jump. Hours of practice were rewarded with a coveted spot on the basketball team, but my position was usually on the bench next to the coach.

One day, Mr. Stargell cornered me and suggested that I might have been built more for wrestling than for basketball. Perhaps he was right, but the high school that I attended did not even have a wrestling team. To my surprise, Mr. Stargell volunteered to help me start one. Given the long odds of a successful basketball career, I began recruiting friends to serve on this hypothetical wrestling team. Although Mr. Stargell knew nothing about wrestling, he was at every practice and at every match during my senior year (Figure 16-2). With his support and encouragement, I never lost a match in the 120-pound weight class, and I could have accepted a wrestling scholarship to college if I had wanted to continue this grueling sport. Never-ending hunger and the prospect of cauliflower ears had convinced me otherwise.

I will always be grateful to Mr. Stargell because he stuck his neck out for me and was directly responsible for the confidence and self-esteem that I developed. The best memories of my high school and college careers were always on some field or court, and athletics has had a profound impact on my life.

Perhaps one of my most important revelations was when I realized that I could have a similar impact on both my own children and other youngsters by accepting the responsibility of coaching their various sports teams. My first job as coach began when my firstborn was four-and-a-half years old, and I coached every single baseball and basketball team through junior high school for each of my five children (Figure 16-3). I looked forward to every season with unbridled enthusiasm as the gloomy Midwestern winters were made tolerable by the sound of balls being dribbled on a hardwood floor in some snow-covered gym (Figure 16-4). Springtime always meant the crack of the bat and the smell of oiled leather. Not only did I coach their recreational teams, I

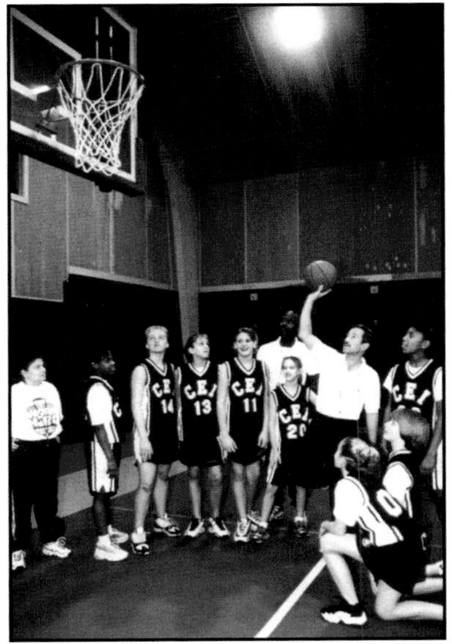

Figure 16-4. Coaching basketball every winter for 3 decades.

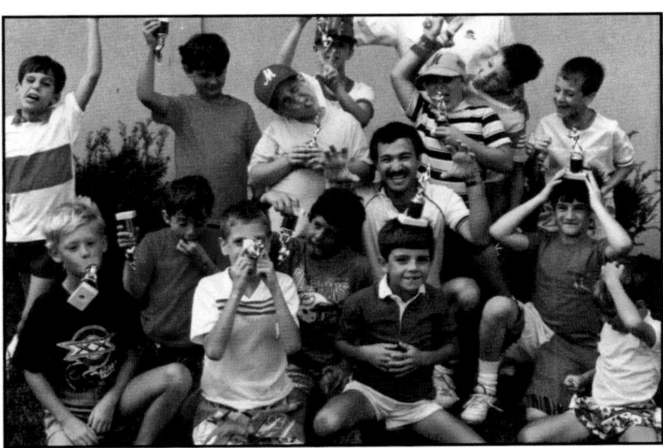

Figure 16-5. My teams won, and we had fun!

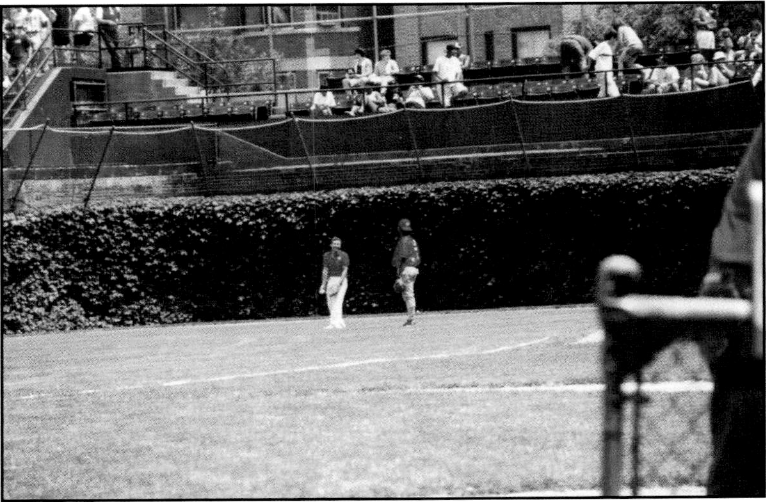

Figure 16-6. Shagging fly balls against the ivy at Wrigley Field during Reds batting practice.

even coached a few of their school teams, and we always had fun (Figure 16-5)! Eventually, I began coaching elite athletes in the Amateur Athletic Union (AAU) programs.

While I read and studied dozens of books on baseball and basketball, I took advantage of a number of friendships with professional athletes. In 1990, I became one of the two team physicians with the Cincinnati Reds and spent a great deal of time shagging balls (Figure 16-6) and talking baseball with managers Lou Piniella and, later, Davey Johnson. Occasionally, I would take my sons into the batting cage (Figure 16-7), where they were on a first-name basis with Mariano Duncan, Hal Morris, Barry Larkin, Reggie Sanders, Glenn Braggs, and other players on the World Championship team. I can vividly remember coaching a 10-year-old team and glancing at my first base coach, Bill Doran, and the third base coach, Billy Hatcher, both major leaguers, and wishing that we had more talent on the other side of the baselines! At the Continental Amateur Baseball Association National Championships in Tarkio, Missouri,

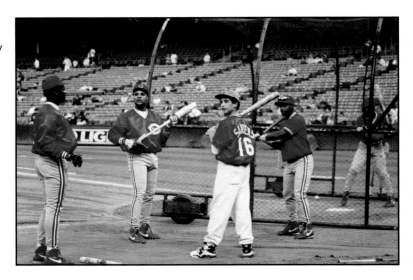

Figure 16-7. Reds players Reggie Sanders, Barry Larkin, and Dion Sanders with Jamey before he decided to study ophthalmology.

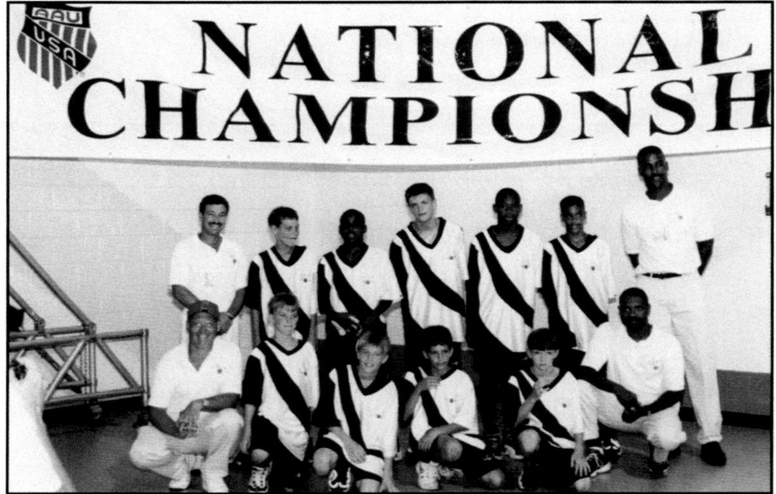

Figure 16-8. My boys achieved a Final Four finish at the AAU National Championships.

I recall noticing that our shortstop, Ricky Bell, was consulting with his father, major league manager Buddy Bell. On that same team was one of my favorite players, whom I coached year after year, Boston Red Sox Hall of Famer, Kevin Youkilis (Note: Kevin is the dignified one next to me in the yellow t-shirt in Figure 16-5). In basketball, I was equally lucky, coaching with Louis Orr, who had played forward for the New York Knicks. I remember taking several teams to the National Championships and was assisted by Stan Kimbrough, an NBA player with the Detroit Pistons. Many of my players went on to receive a free college education.

All in all, I calculated that I must have coached about 70 teams, most of which seemed to overachieve, a reflection of our preparedness. For example, we had seven consecutive Ohio State AAU basketball Championships and a Final Four finish for both boys (Figure 16-8) and girls (Figure 16-9) at the National Championships held in Disney World. I just do not think that there could have been anything more fun than watching these youngsters develop as players while becoming fast friends.

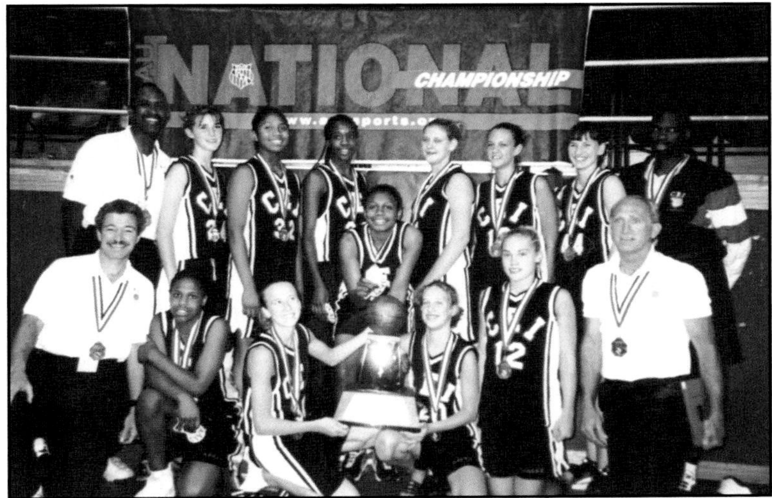

Figure 16-9. My girls' team also finished in the Final Four at the "big dance."

Are kids too young to compete?

Basketball at heart of Indian Hill rift

BY JANET C. WETZEL
The Cincinnati Enquirer

INDIAN HILL — The issue of whether kindergartners, first- and second-graders should be allowed to play competitive basketball has residents and officials in the Indian Hill Recreation Commission at odds.

Bob Osher wants to see a change in the way the youth basketball program is run. When Osher's son, Jon, then a first-grader, wanted to play basketball. He formed a team and asked the recreation commission to help.

Osher said not only did Alley refuse to support the effort, but the commission would not allow the team gym time to practice, would not notify parents that there was an alternative program available, and refused to let the new team wear commission uniforms or use the Indian Hill name.

"We had to split out," of the Queen City Basketball League and

> "They did a disservice to the community, the children and the families by discontinuing the basketball program for those children."
>
> **Nick Bagnoli**

gram from about 85 to more tha 325 children.

Alley said it "boils down t serving the most people, and think the instructional program ha served the most people in the wa they want to be served." Man communities do not have competi tive K-2 basketball, he said.

Steve Smith, owner/director o the Queen City Basketball League which represents teams from 5 Greater Cincinnati communities agreed, but said more communitie are adding programs for the youn

Figure 16-10. Controversy makes the news. Am I teaching kids to compete too young?

Coaching has the potential to impact our future generations, and I cannot think of a better way for a young person to learn so many important values in life. Success does not come by accident; it comes from hard work. Effort and preparation always pay dividends. Moreover, there is no better place to learn the concept of team and the responsibility that each player has to one another. The art of both winning and losing with dignity are critical lessons that last a lifetime.

When we moved into our community, I attempted to initiate a youth sports program for young primary school children. A spirited debate erupted, and I was criticized in the newspaper for allegedly igniting competitive fires at too young an age (Figure 16-10). Those who were most critical really missed the point. When you teach a youngster to perform a sport well, he or she is inevitably praised by his or her peers. The child likes this feeling, which raises self-esteem and confidence. He or she wants to engage in this activity even more, and, not unexpectedly, improvement continues. More praise follows, and both self-esteem and confidence continue to escalate. It is a very positive, self-propagating cycle.

These benefits and values are not limited to children. Senator Bill Bradley, a Rhodes Scholar and former New York Knicks standout, authored a book entitled *The Values of the Game*. I share his belief that the lessons learned on the basketball court apply to most of life's situations (Figure 16-11). For example, many of the physicians whom I hired were asked to participate in

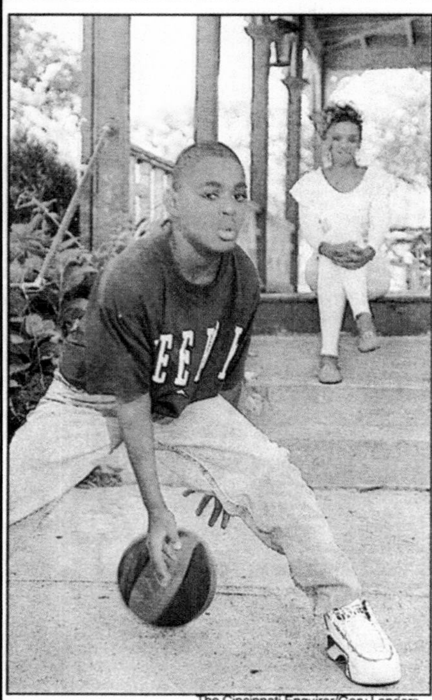

The Cincinnati Enquirer/Gary Landers

John Brown was a member of the Ohio AAU basketball team that placed third at the national tournament. Iva Brown is in the background.

Coach teaches boy about life through basketball

He is waiting in front of the big old house in Bond Hill, an 11-year-old wearing size-10 Converse high tops, bouncing a basketball off the cracked sidewalk.

Slap-slap-slap.

John Brown has oversized hands that make the ball do his bidding. Behind his back. Between his legs. Back and forth, easy as breathing. Slap-slap-slap.

"You John?" I ask.

"Yup," he says.

"You play a little ball?"

"Some."

John Brown played on a team of local 11-year-olds that just finished third in the national AAU basketball tournament. It's believed to be the best an Ohio team has ever done in that event. They reached the semifinals because John banked in a fadeaway jumper as time expired. But that's hardly important.

Here's what is:

John's mother Iva is in the house, with her parents and John's cousin, in a living room covered in pictures of family. Iva says, "Basketball has been a

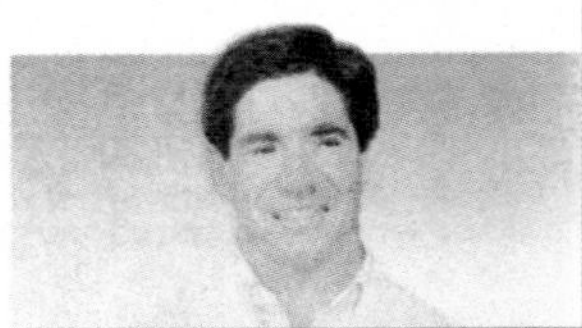

PAUL DAUGHERTY

self-esteem builder for John. If he feels good about himself, it will make him a better person all around."

On the phone the night before, Iva fought tears. John's coach, Bob Osher, called her to say I'd be coming to talk to John. "You know how proud we all are of your son," Osher said, "how hard he has worked to become a better player and person.

"It'd be a feather in his cap to be mentioned in the newspaper, and lord knows, he deserves it," Osher said.

Now, the kid in the big shoes tosses a tape in the VCR. It replays a story a local TV station

(Please see DAUGHERTY, Page C15)

Figure 16-11. Front page story in the Cincinnati Enquirer reflects the values of the game.

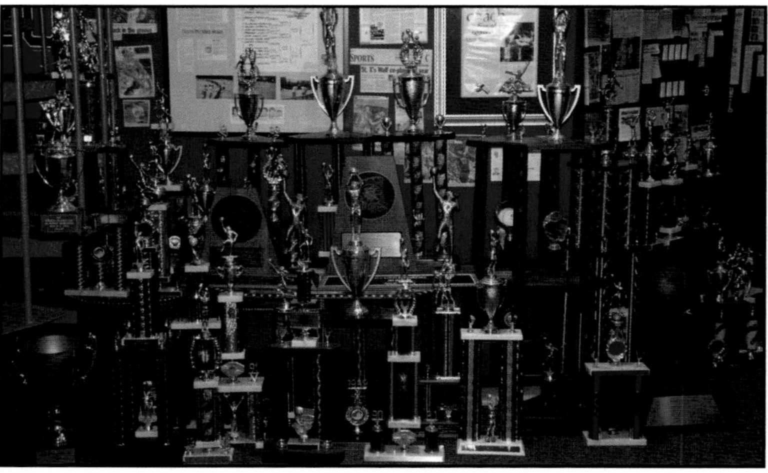

Figure 16-12. Ain't no art in our house!

a sporting event during their interview. If, during a tennis match, the physician gave every shot his or her best effort and demonstrated integrity by calling any ball that was close "in," he or she was probably cut from the right fabric to succeed in our organization.

When we built our home, it was not necessary to invest in decorative art. Instead of art, there are a plethora of team trophies, which trigger some of the greatest memories of my life (Figure 16-12). There is one trophy that means a little more than all of the rest, Ohio Coach of

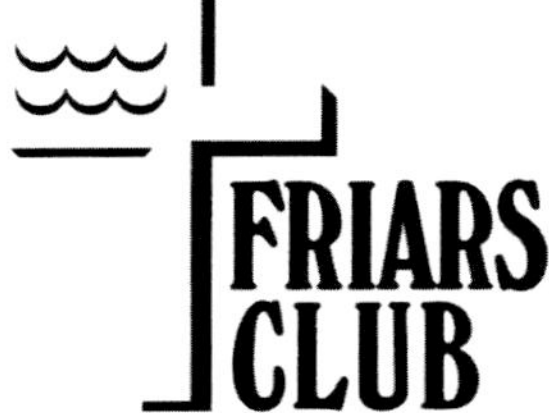

You Are Cordially Invited To Attend

FRIARS CLUB
THIRTY-FIFTH ANNUAL
COMMUNITY DINNER

THE COACH OF THE YEAR AWARD:
Recipient: BOB OSHER

MASTER OF CEREMONIES:
ROB BRAUN

COCKTAIL HOUR: 6:00 p.m.
DINNER and PROGRAM: 7:00 p.m.

Black Tie Optional

Figure 16-13. This honor was especially meaningful.

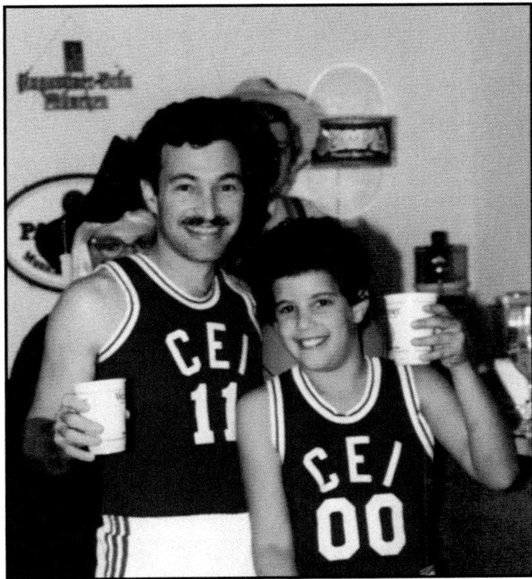

Figure 16-14. Here's to the best of times! Father and son celebrate Cincinnati Eye Institute's undefeated basketball season.

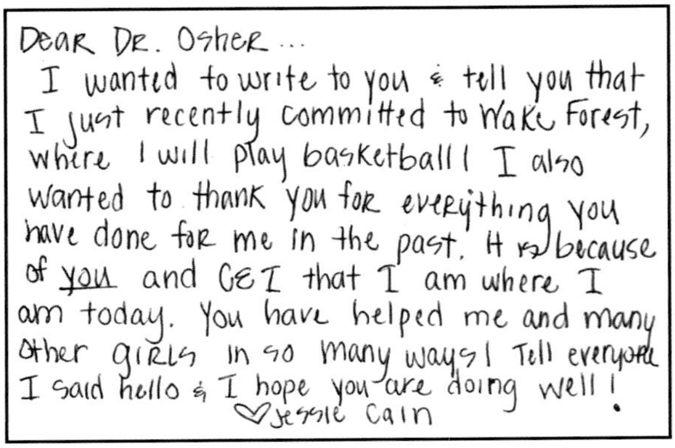

Dear Dr. Osher...
I wanted to write to you & tell you that I just recently committed to Wake Forest, where I will play basketball! I also wanted to thank you for everything you have done for me in the past. It is because of you and CEI that I am where I am today. You have helped me and many other girls in so many ways! Tell everyone I said hello & I hope you are doing well!
♥Jessie Cain

Figure 16-15. It is difficult to express how deep these letters touch me.

the Year from the Friars Club, an inner-city organization that specializes in saving troubled kids (Figure 16-13). It reminds me that a season is not measured by the number of wins, but rather by the personal growth of the players.

It may sound selfish, but I could not think of a better way to derive many hours of pleasure with my own children than getting immersed in their recreational activities. From their diaper days onward, we played catch together and worked on developing their athletic skills. Not only did I cherish every moment with my own children (Figure 16-14), I treasured participating in the development of many fine young athletes (Figure 16-15). Can you imagine the thrill of learning that little Kevin Youkilis was drafted by the Boston Red Sox, received a Gold Glove, was voted three times by the fans to the All Star team, and is now in the Red Sox Hall of Fame (Figure 16-16)? How exciting that little Josh and Johnny were each named Ohio Basketball

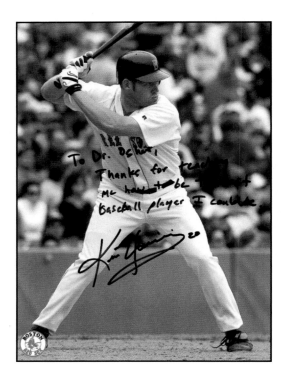

Figure 16-16. Do you want to see a sentimental old man tear up? Check out this "Thank you" from Boston All-Star Kevin Youkilis.

Player of the Year, while Lesslee, Desi, and Diondra also received the same title for girls' high school basketball. Myia even reached the NCAA finals. Do you want to feel really, really good? Commit yourself to working with our next generation, and it may even keep you young a bit longer while you are having the time of your life!

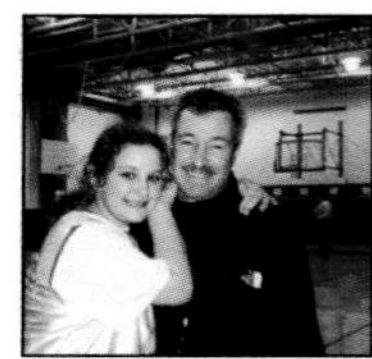

CHAPTER 17

Adventure!

Every person should have the opportunity to experience the exhilaration of pure adventure. It is difficult to define the meaning of adventure, as it certainly differs from individual to individual. Yet, it must be an activity that is vastly different from the daily routine. Adventure creates anticipation; its execution is adrenaline provoking, and when completed, it provides a pleasurable memory. These would include activities like mountain climbing, kayaking, scuba diving, dirt biking, skiing, whitewater rafting, etc. These diversions may be the subject around which one plans a vacation, and financial resources are often necessary. Yet, I believe that achieving complete self-Contentment often means extracting every bit of enjoyment and excitement that is available on God's magnificent playground.

I feel very fortunate to have been invited to speak in so many unusual places around the world. These invitations have often resulted in fantastic adventures. Following a lecture to the Brazilian Cataract Society, I disappeared into the Amazon for several days, cutting a path through the rain forest with a machete (Figure 17-1) and making new acquaintances when I emerged (Figure 17-2). Traversing the Great Wall of China was an exhilarating experience (Figure 17-3), as was attempting to sprint to the top of Ayer's Rock in Australia (Figure 17-4). I have enjoyed trying to land game fish on light tackle in the fast-moving waters in South America (Figure 17-5) or trying to catch barramundi while avoiding the flesh-eating, 25-foot, salt water crocodiles in the northern wilderness of Australia. Diving in the Caribbean, Bali, or off the Great Barrier Reef were incredible excursions (Figure 17-6), especially when encountering submarine-sized bronze whaler and bull sharks.

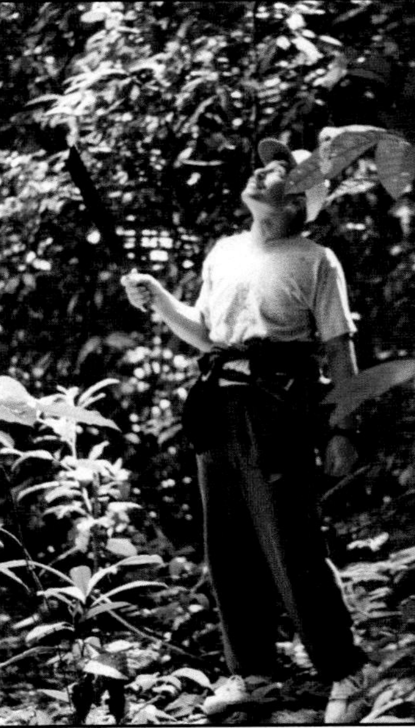

Figure 17-1. Hacking through the rainforest in the Amazon.

Osher RH. *The Real ABCs: A Surgeon's Analysis and a Father's Legacy, Second Edition* (pp 77-83).

Figure 17-2. Are you sure it doesn't bite?

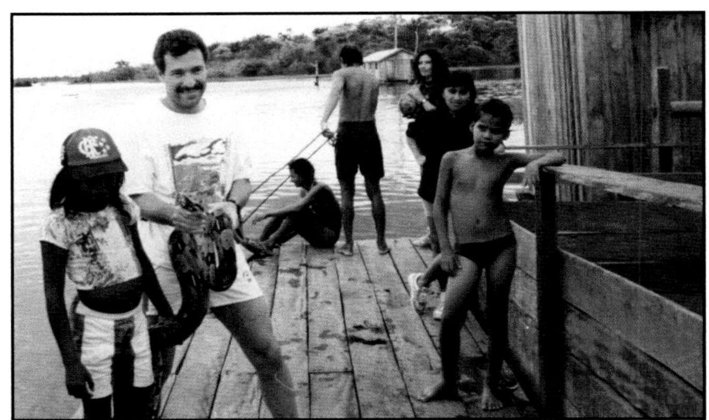

Figure 17-3. Experiencing the Great Wall of China.

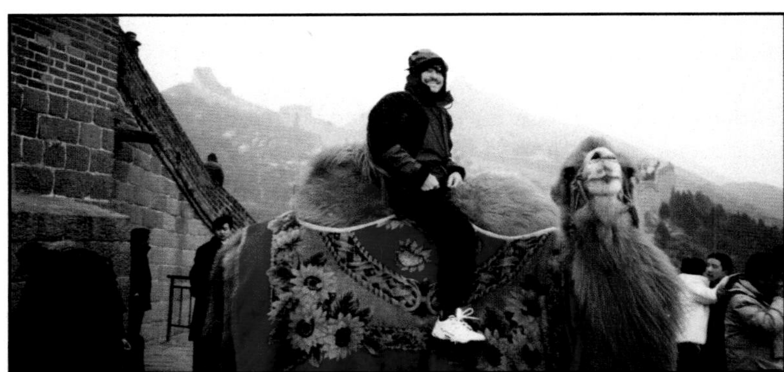

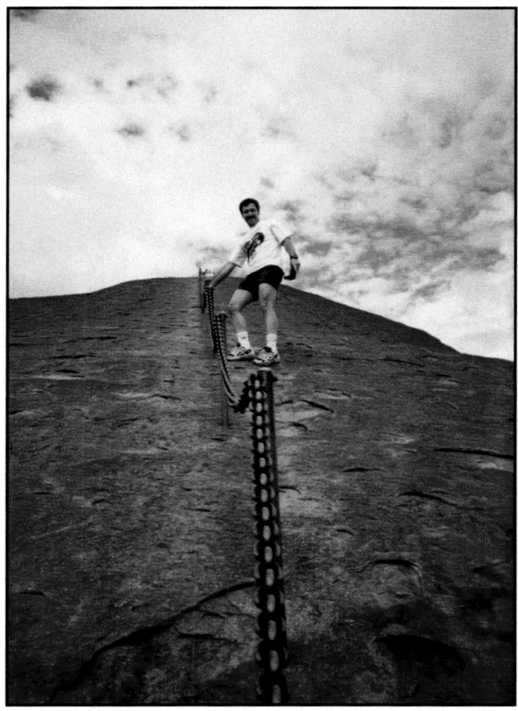

Figure 17-4. Sprinting to the top of Ayer's Rock in Australia.

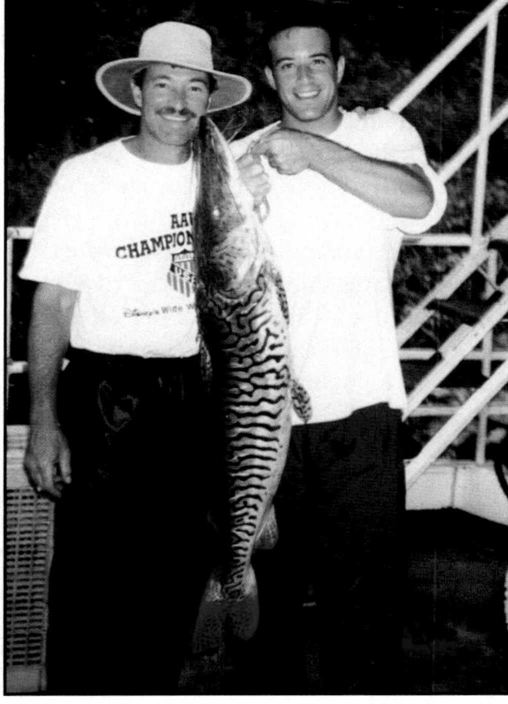

Figure 17-5. Game fishing in South America with my son, Jeff.

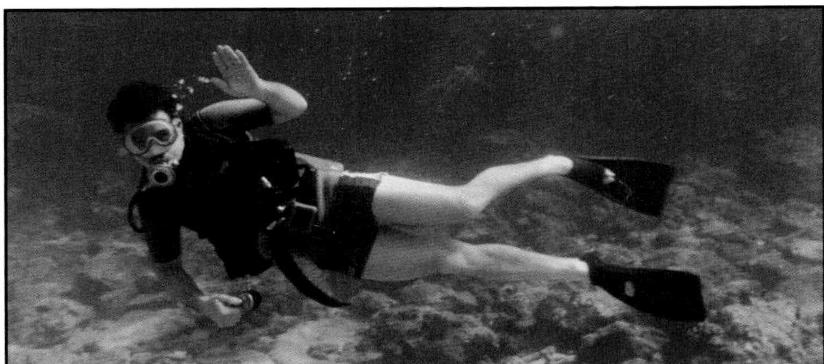

Figure 17-6. No pagers or cell phones allowed!

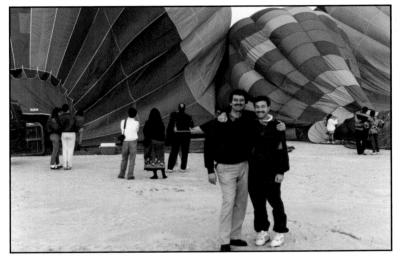

Figure 17-7. Ballooning with famous German surgeon, Thomas Neuhann, MD.

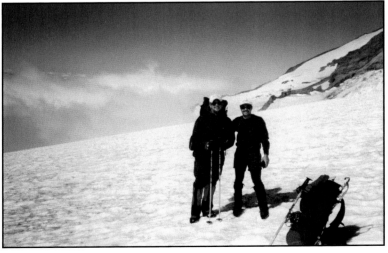

Figure 17-8. Above the clouds climbing Mount Rainier with Jamey.

Who would have thought that ballooning along the coast or over the Alps could be so much fun (Figure 17-7)? Climbing Mount Rainier at 2:00 am with an ice axe to arrest a fall into a bottomless crevasse while tied with a rope to my son was unforgettable (Figure 17-8).

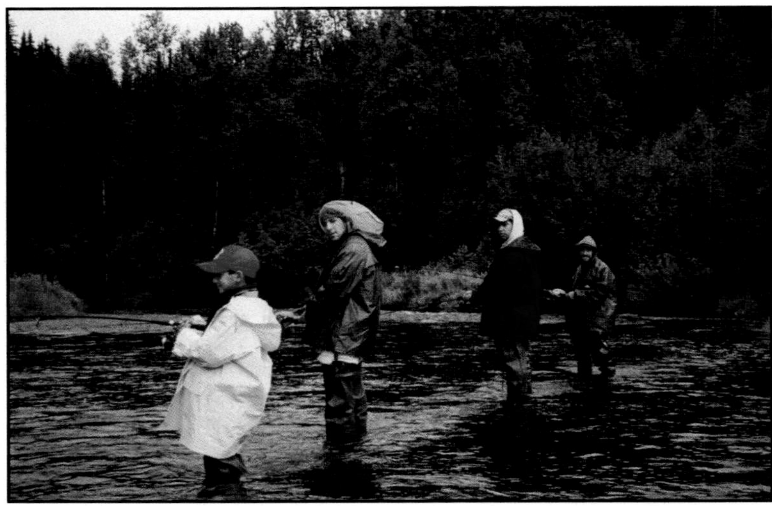

Figure 17-9. Salmon fishing in Alaska with my boys, Jon, Jeff, and Jamey.

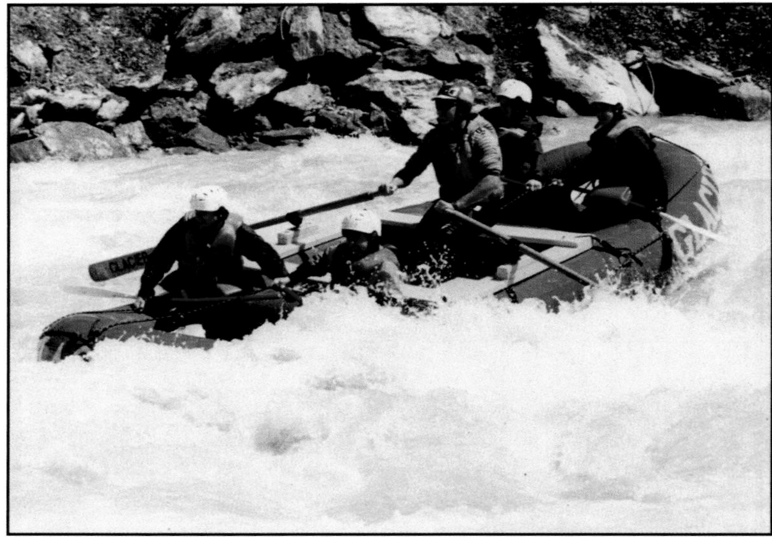

Figure 17-10. Whitewater rafting on the Bow River, hoping not to lose a kid!

Fishing with my boys for salmon in grizzly bear territory in Alaska (Figure 17-9), bike racing around a 19-mile island in the Pacific, and whitewater rafting in the Canadian Rockies (Figure 17-10) were great adventures. I will never forget kayaking down the Salt River in Arizona with Jenny (Figure 17-11), ziplining upside down with Debbie in Costa Rica (Figure 17-12), and safariing with family in South Africa (Figure 17-13). Even climbing the Sydney Bridge over the Opera House with Barbara and our two daughters as we clung to each other against a 40-MPH headwind was adrenalizing (Figure 17-14)! Flying on an ultralight (basically a chair, wing, and fan) over Victoria Falls in Zambia did not cure my acrophobia (Figure 17-15), and just try serenading a cobra in India (Figure 17-16)!

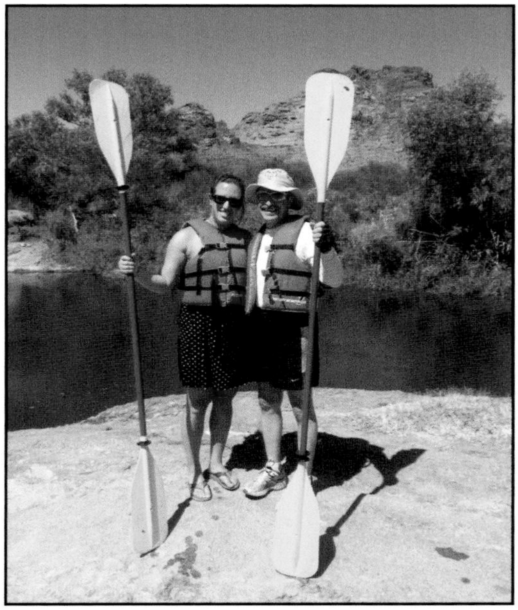
Figure 17-11. Kayaking with Jenny was a blast!

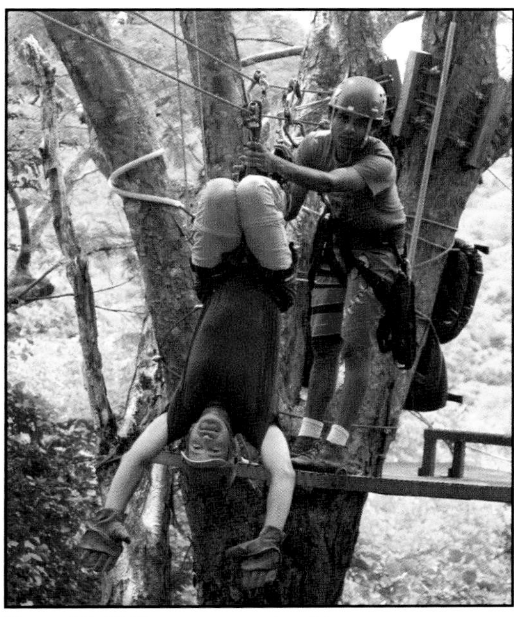
Figure 17-12. Here comes my lunch!

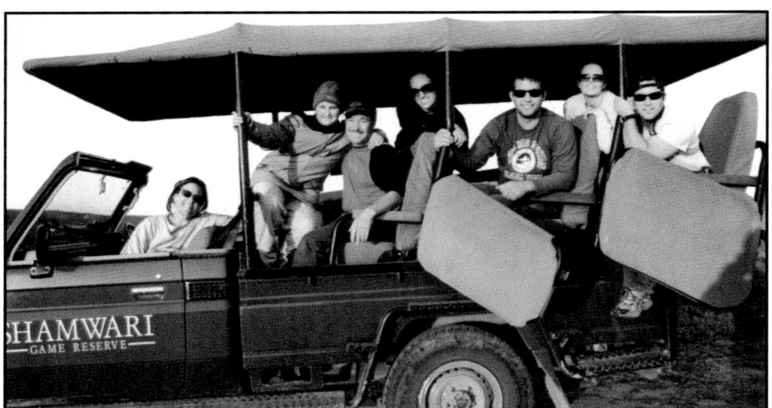

Figure 17-13. After lecturing in Cape Town, my family loved our first safari.

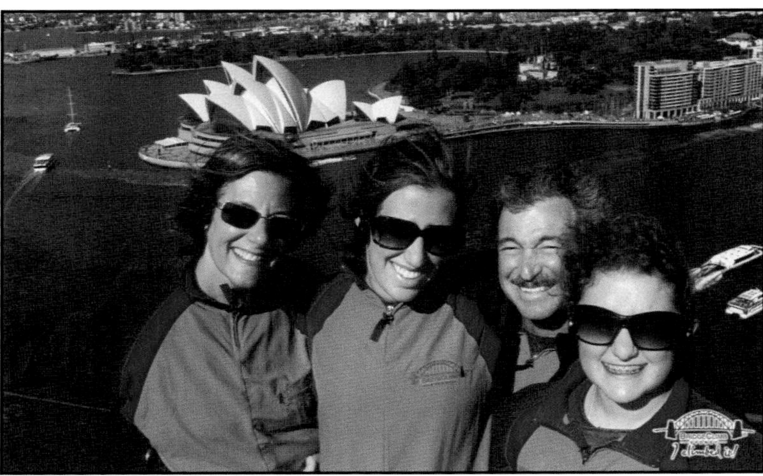
Figure 17-14. Climbing the Bay Bridge high above the Sydney Opera House in gale-force winds with Barb, Jenny, and Jessie.

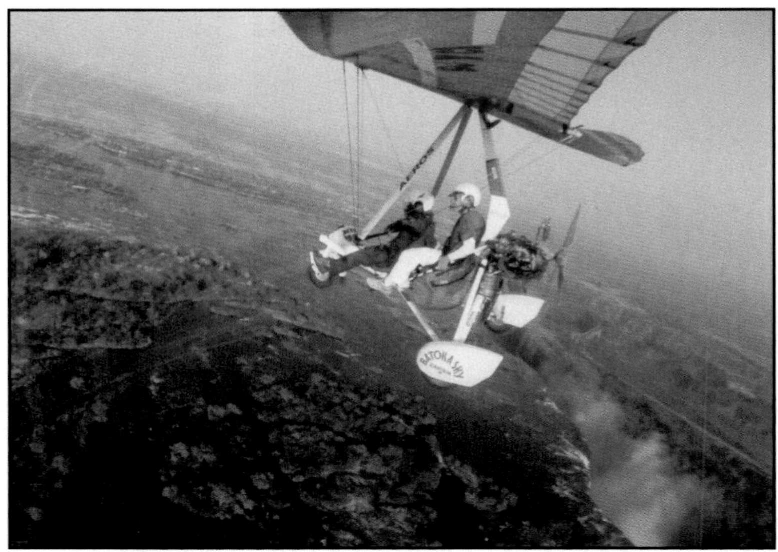

Figure 17-15. My first and last ultralight over Victoria Falls in Zimbabwe.

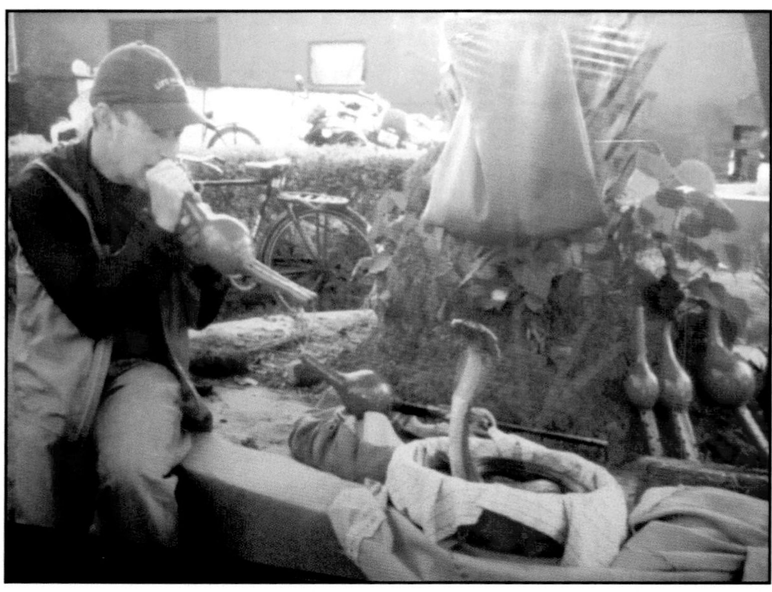

Figure 17-16. Any last requests?

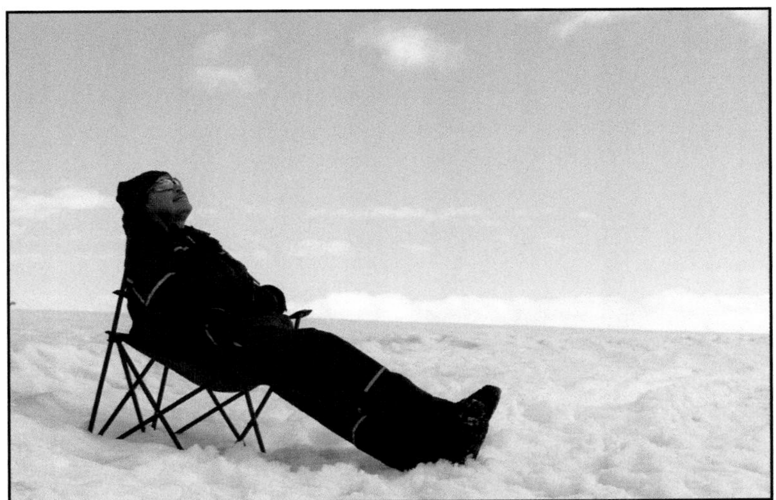

Figure 17-17. Glacier napping—wake me up before nightfall.

The list of adventures is truly infinite, but each one of us is capable of "spicing up" our lives and escaping from the occasional rut of our daily routine. The nature of the adventure certainly varies. For example, I have little desire to jump out of a plane with a parachute attached to my back, nor do I wish to leap off a cliff in Rio with a pair of "wings" attached to my arms. However, I was willing to try napping on a glacier in Iceland (Figure 17-17). I have friends who look forward to their annual camping trip, and still others who cannot wait to hit the ski slopes every Christmas. The bottom line is that each of these adventures represents a personal accomplishment in itself and should be rightfully included in the record of our lifetime Achievements.

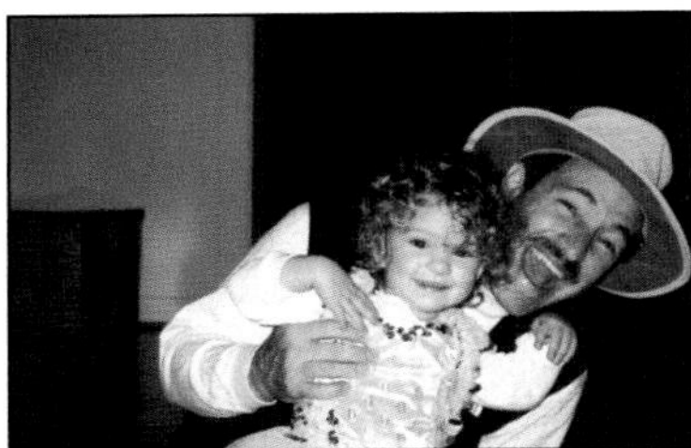

CHAPTER 18

Enjoying the Outdoors
(God's Playground)

While adventure should be exhilarating, as described in the previous chapter, the simple enjoyment of the outdoors represents a more sedate and less expensive luxury. All that I can remember about my childhood in Cincinnati, Ohio was that the winters were extremely cold and my hands were always frostbitten. It got worse during medical school in Rochester, New York, where I learned to value the 1 day of summer. During my residency training, I had the opportunity to experience never-ending Miami, Florida summers, during which time I was always sweating and seeking the miracles of modern air conditioning. Then, after my diagnosis of cancer, my awareness and appreciation of the outdoors changed dramatically, and I began to enjoy the sights and sounds of nature. While the sight of feeding caimans, the sound of the shrill cry of a spider monkey, and the wiry feel of a tarantula in the Amazon can get anyone's attention (Figure 18-1), I realized that one does not have to travel very far to feel the same euphoria. In fact, just 1 mile from my home, I discovered a small river into which I could throw a kayak several times per week and paddle through rapids for several miles without encountering another soul. It is incredibly satisfying to observe the wildlife while kayaking down the river. What a terrific cure for a stressful day (Figure 18-2)!

It took more than 5 decades and a life-threatening diagnosis to finally experience the joy that comes from inhaling nature's beauty. I relish the colorful sunsets and the star-filled skies when walking the dog at night. I marvel at the tapestry of colors as the trees transition from summer to fall (Figure 18-3). I am mesmerized by the flight of the red-tailed hawk that glides effortlessly through the air just before sundown. I am captivated by the family of red foxes that saunter across the golf course at dusk, and every butterfly must be photographed (Figure 18-4).

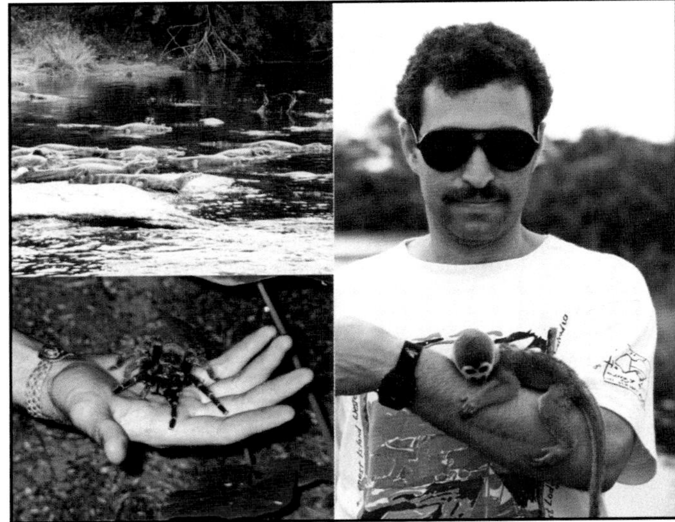

Figure 18-1. These critters will get your attention!

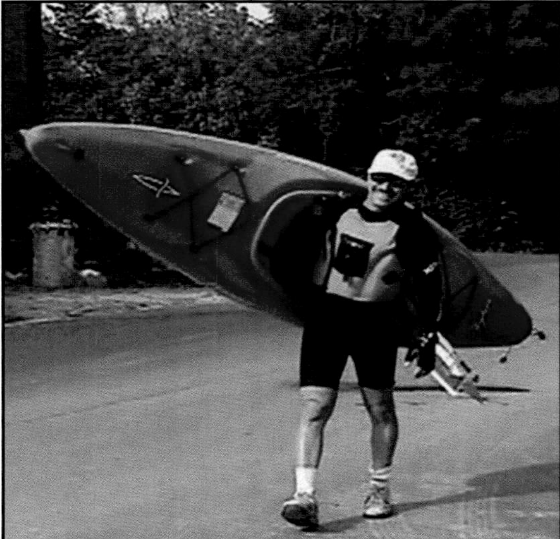

Figure 18-2. Kayaking is a magical way to end a stressful day.

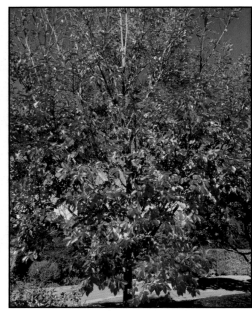

Figure 18-3. These trees look like they were imported from another planet!

Figure 18-4. Monarchs: mandatory photographic opportunity.

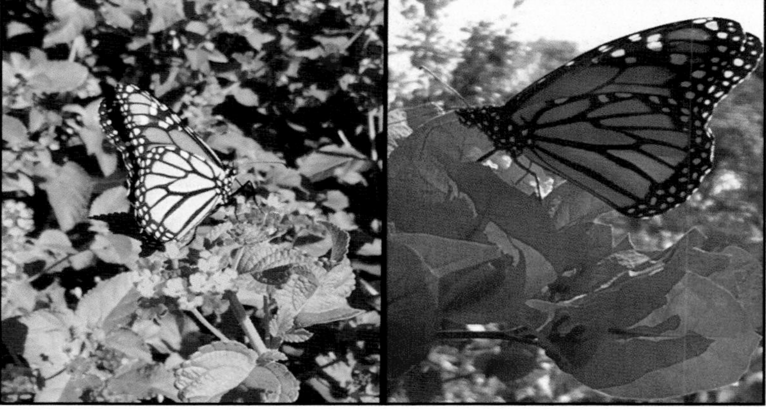

Since my brush with death, I seem to treasure not only animal life, but all living things. My home is surrounded by spectacular gardens that I planted after reading several books about the perennials and shrubs that flourish in our region (Figures 18-5 and 18-6). I memorized the flowering characteristics, colors, heights, bloom seasons, soil types, amount of sunlight required, and where each plant would thrive in relation to other plants. What had always seemed like a boring, sedate hobby became very vibrant the more knowledgeable I became. When the bulbs and flowers began to explode in color, it was like I had created an artistic masterpiece (Figure 18-7)! An additional benefit was that the blooms seemed to welcome a legion of colorful songbirds and butterflies, each a small but magnificent celebration of life.

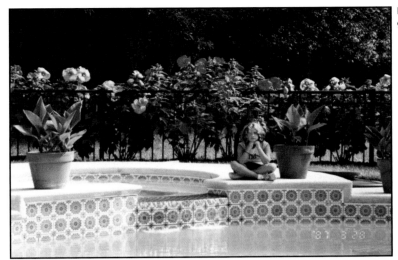

Figure 18-5. Turns out that gardening is very relaxing...

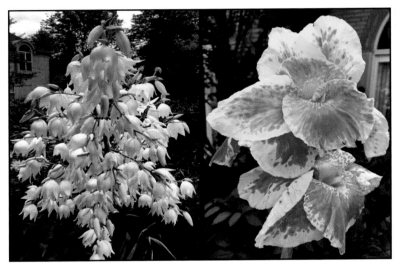

Figure 18-6. ...and quite spectacular!

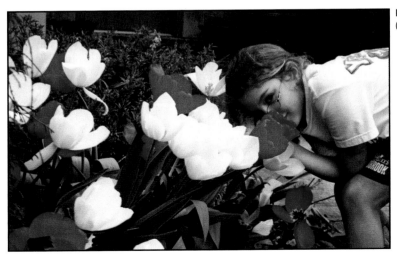

Figure 18-7. Beautiful, isn't she (Jessie)...my flowers are too!

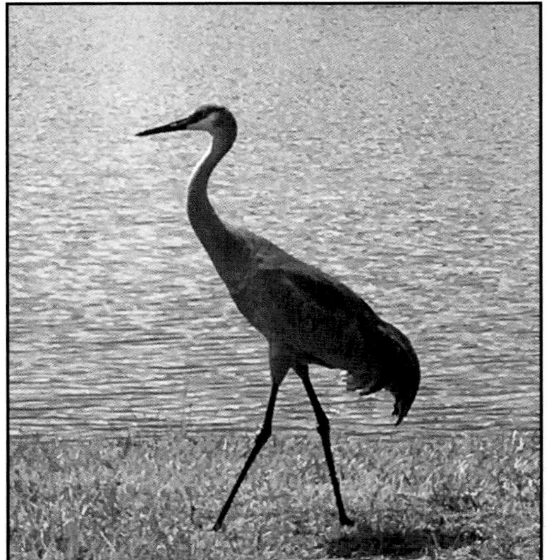

Figure 18-8. Red-headed sandhill crane.

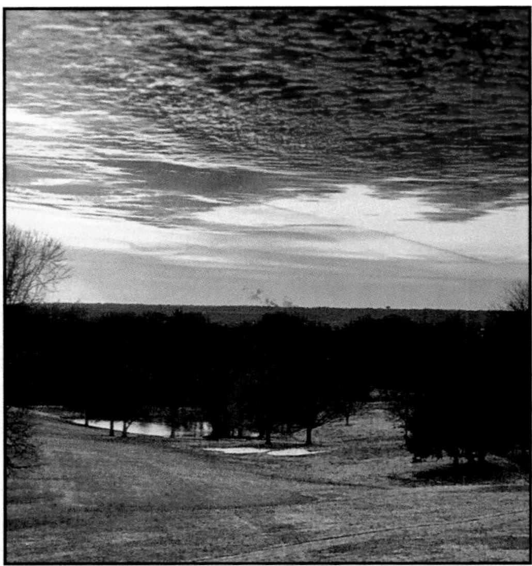

Figure 18-9. Majestic sunset rewards the last golfer of the course.

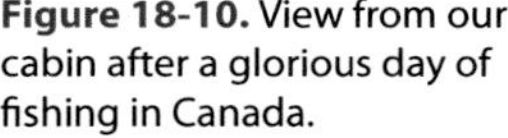

Figure 18-10. View from our cabin after a glorious day of fishing in Canada.

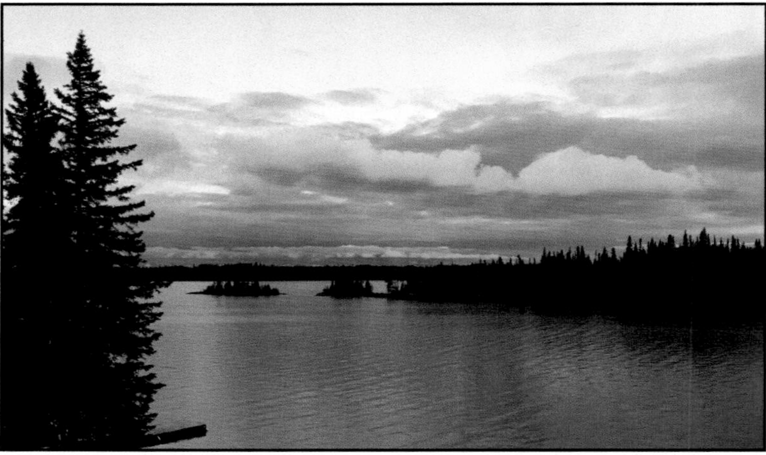

I believe that if one takes the time to learn about flowers, trees, birds, butterflies, and the many constituents of the outdoors, he or she will be rewarded by a heightened sense of awareness and appreciation of the spectrum of miracles we call *nature*. Never again will I miss or take for granted the extraordinary colors of the critters (Figure 18-8), sunsets (Figure 18-9), landscapes (Figure 18-10), and seasons that serve to make life so much more enchanting. It's all right there, no admission necessary. Just open your eyes…and enjoy!

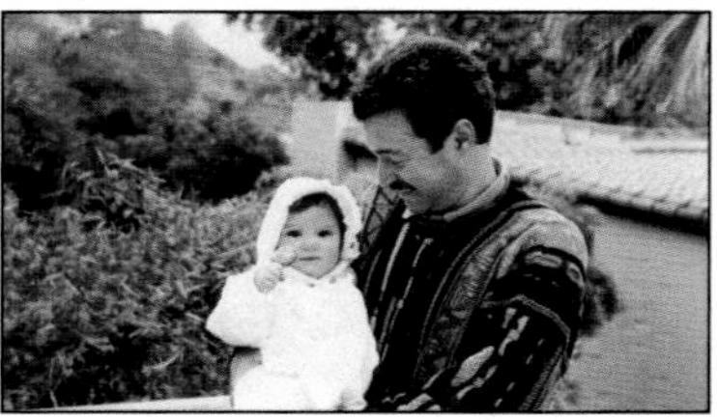

CHAPTER 19

Top Priority

Family!

I am certain that if all American adults were surveyed and asked, "What is the single most important thing in your life?" the overwhelming majority would answer emphatically, "Family!" There might be a few individuals who would volunteer other answers like wealth, prestige, fame, health, etc, but our genetic constitution guarantees a high degree of attention devoted to the bond between parent and child. Moreover, if the survey included a question soliciting the key to our future, again, the answer would be, "Our children." Then, how ironic is it that the typical high school or college graduate can speak a foreign language, solve an algebraic equation, or recite a portion of the Gettysburg Address, but very few have any clue about how to raise a family or lead our children in the right direction? I confess to being a member of the uneducated group.

While each of us may have unwavering convictions with respect to our own values, how can we expect our offspring to inherit these ideals? Will it pass on by luck, by osmosis, or by the genetic code? Doubtful. We have to work just as hard, if not harder, toward achieving a well-balanced child as we work toward any major achievement in our career. I wish I could hit reverse and do this all over again.

There is little time to get the job done correctly. The kids are usually in school, and we are usually at work. Then, the kids are playing with their friends and we are pursuing our own recreational interests. When the kids become mature enough that we really enjoy their company, they have their own social agenda with little time for their parents. In the blink of an eye, they are off to college, and soon after, beginning to raise a family of their own. Everything happens way too fast.

I was incredibly lucky to be born into a family surrounded by love and support from my mother, father, sister, and brother (Figure 19-1). As the result, we all turned out pretty well. My sister, Nancy, a registered nurse, started a wonderful program to help children in Rwanda in East Africa called *Books and Beyond* in partnership with Indiana University in Bloomington. She also brought the miracle of drinkable water to small villages in need of a well. She married the multi-talented Michael Uslan, who is the executive producer of the incredibly popular *Batman* movies. My brother, Sandy, became a respected gynecology surgeon who popularized laparoscopy in the Midwest. To the best of my knowledge, none of us have ever served time, even though on occasion we have been tempted to murder one another!

Admittedly, I have made more than my fair share of mistakes raising my own children, and despite my blunders, each of my kids is grounded, happy, confident, and successful. Jeff is a highly-respected hedge-fund manager in San Francisco and one heck of a baseball coach.

Osher RH. *The Real ABCs: A Surgeon's Analysis and a Father's Legacy, Second Edition* (pp 89-93).

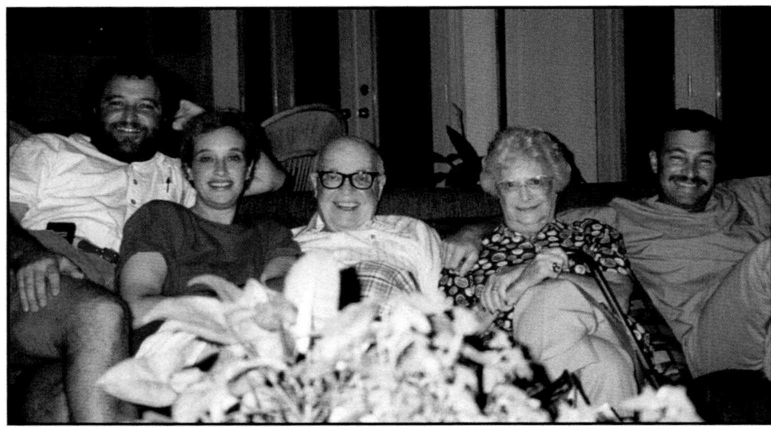
Figure 19-1. Brother, Sandy; sister, Nancy; Dad; and Mom.

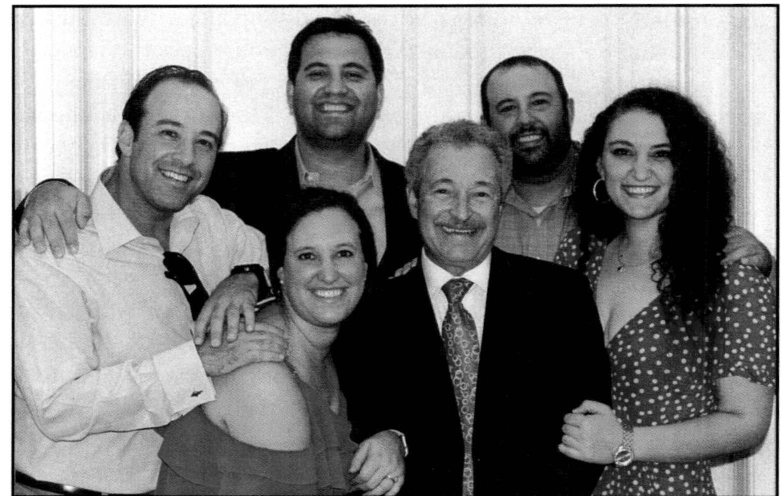
Figure 19-2. Surrounded by the Osher "Pride"—sons Jeff, Jon, and Jamey, and daughters Jenny and Jessie.

Jamey is an outstanding retinal specialist at CEI. Jon owns a successful real estate company buying, selling, and managing rental properties. Jenny is a fabulous nurse. Jessie is an exceptional student at Clemson (Figure 19-2). Their personalities are different not only from mine, but also from each other. Sometimes, it is difficult to believe that they share the same gene pool! Nevertheless, I am convinced that there are several universal key principles and basic practices that have had a positive effect on each child's development.

First, from the day that each of our children was born, we have emphasized that Mom and Dad would stand by them under any circumstances. This does not mean that we would condone an error in judgement any more than we would overlook a mischievous or dishonest act. What it does mean, however, is that no matter how great the magnitude of their problem, we will always try to help them in difficult times. In every family, there are going to be some difficult times—guaranteed!

Second, we have talked openly with our children about values. While we may have been guilty of sending mixed signals when it came to discipline, responsibility, time management, etc, there was no ambiguity regarding what is right and what is wrong. Certainly, all kids are going to occasionally test and break the rules (just like their parents did), and ours have been no exception, but when it comes to matters of integrity and loyalty to each other, the message has been crystal clear. It makes me proud that all five children are as tight as a band of thieves.

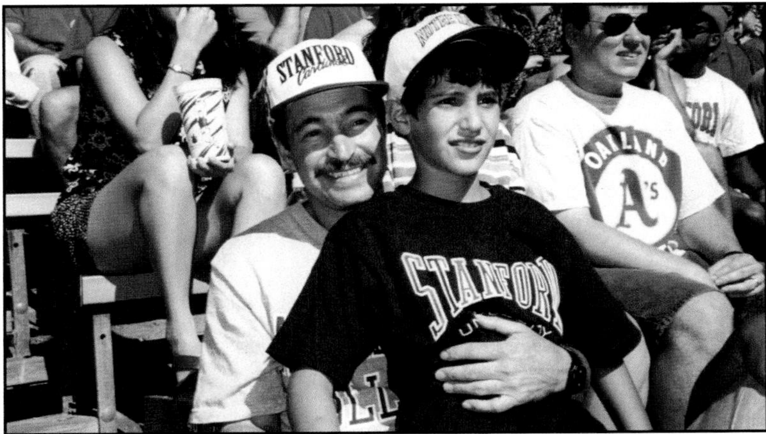

Figure 19-3. Following a lecture at Stanford, Jon and I enjoy a football game together.

Third, I strongly believe in giving each child a head start. Children are like sponges, and they can absorb practically anything that is thrown their way. Each of our children was reading by age 3 and could understand square roots by age 5. By age 6, each could throw, catch, hit, dribble, and shoot. It is my belief that when you give your child a running start, he or she will eventually be judged positively by their peers and praised, which feels very good inside. As a result of this positive feedback, the child wants to engage in the activity at every opportunity, and the additional practice pays off. The level of competence continues to improve, and the praise continues to follow. Both self-esteem and confidence grow. Although this cycle applies to virtually any activity, it is especially applicable and beneficial in sports because of the emphasis that our society places on youth athletics. Daughters, Jen and Jessie, have enjoyed success competing in sports with the boys in their classes and have developed a great deal of self-confidence. Our sons, Jeff, Jamey, and Jon, were especially accomplished in athletics, and this proficiency has carried into their professional careers.

Fourth, I experimented with an idea that has paid big dividends in terms of quality time. Since I was often invited out of town to speak to ophthalmology societies, rather than endure time away from the kids, I tried to take one child with me as often as possible. We would be able to enjoy the plane ride to and from the venue, as well as the time before and after my lecture (Figure 19-3). Without interruptions or distractions from my office, it was special time reserved for the two of us. Some of my favorite memories originated during these weekend trips. I can vividly recall an invitation to speak to the ophthalmology residents at the prestigious Wilmer Institute at Johns Hopkins in Baltimore, Maryland. After several hours of lecturing early in the morning, the lights came on and the moderator announced that it was time for a brief coffee break. Everyone arose from their chairs and made their way up the stadium stairs to the refreshment area, where a large pot of coffee was brewing adjacent to an even larger tray of donuts. Mysteriously, each of the approximately 50 donuts had a single bite missing! I was embarrassed to discover my 6-year-old son beneath the table with a devious smile on his otherwise angelic face.

Another story comes to mind, when I took two of my young boys with me for a lecture to the Virginia Ophthalmology Society in Norfolk. I happened to be wearing very tight pants, which abruptly split upon bending over just before the lecture began. I asked for the lights to be turned down, and I would have managed to avoid any attention, had both boys not found the red and green laser pointers. For the next hour, they irradiated my groin, causing the broken zipper to light up like a Christmas tree. I would not trade these memories for anything, although I was tempted to trade two kids!

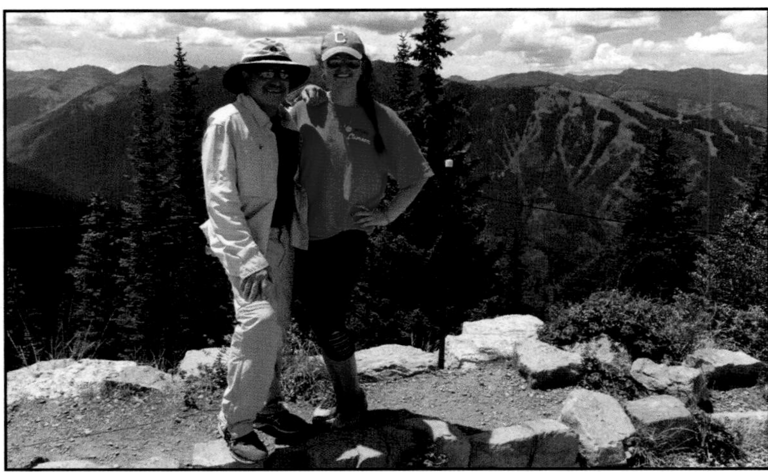

Figure 19-4. Hiking up some mountain in Aspen with Jessie.

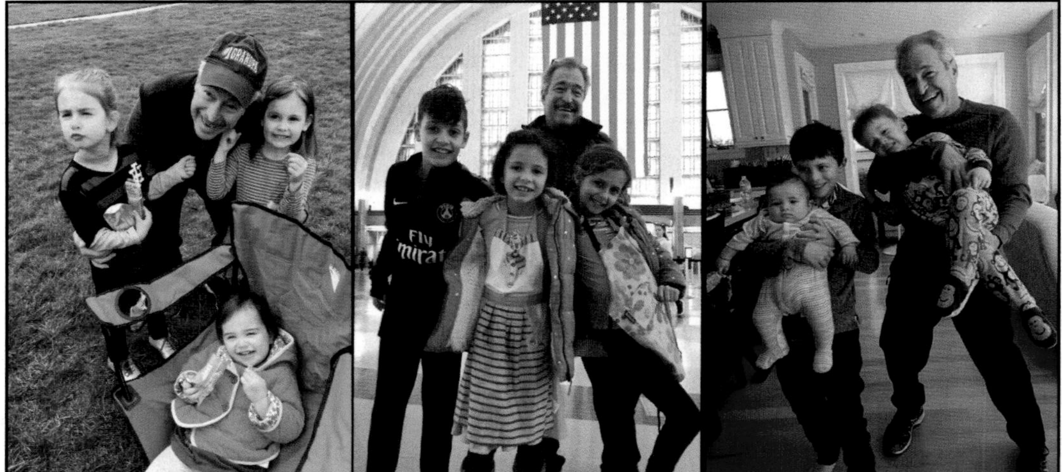

Figure 19-5. Grandchildren—the best!

As I age, spending precious time with a child or grandchild becomes even more rewarding. When possible, I make a special effort to schedule a quick trip or a long weekend not linked to a lecture (Figure 19-4), and I am spending more and more quality time with grandchildren (Figure 19-5). As a senior citizen, I expect my vision to begin to deteriorate, yet what is really important in life is becoming clearer every day (Figure 19-6).

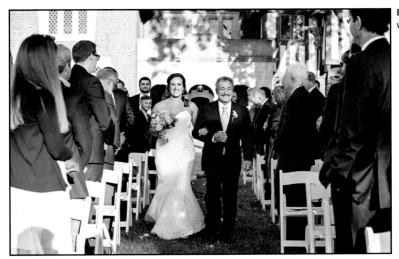

Figure 19-6. My favorite walk with Jenny.

One final thought: I have consistently verbalized my love for each of our children. In our tough-guy society, it may be more difficult for many fathers to express affection toward their children, especially toward their sons. Yet, I really do not want my children to think of me as a "Rock of Gibraltar." It is far more important that they are the recipients of unconditional love, supported by words and confirmed by actions. Their mother, Barb, has been really exceptional and still reaps the rewards for showering the kids with affection from the day they were born. Sure, there are times when I would like to strangle each child, but down deep where it counts, they know that Dad loves them with every fiber of his being.

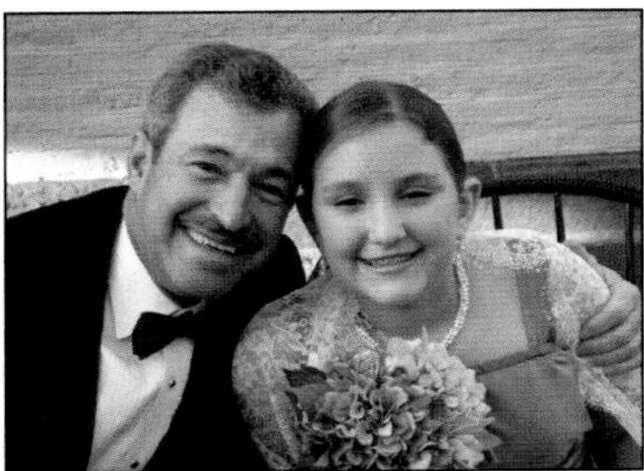

CHAPTER 20

Good Friends

I have always been a lucky man. One of the primary reasons is that I have had a handful of very good friends. Not many, I should add, but the few that I have are real gems. The most precious friendships are the ones that date back to childhood (Figure 20-1). It is amazing that I could move away for a decade and the friendships endure. When I returned to Cincinnati, Ohio, the relationships picked up right where they left off!

While comfortable with people, I never considered myself to be much of a social creature. In fact, I rather enjoy and value my solitude when I am running, biking, kayaking, or just listening to music while working on my surgery charts after everyone is asleep. Yet, there is truth to the saying, "No man is an island."* We really need to be connected to friends and family in order to derive the greatest enjoyment from our lives.

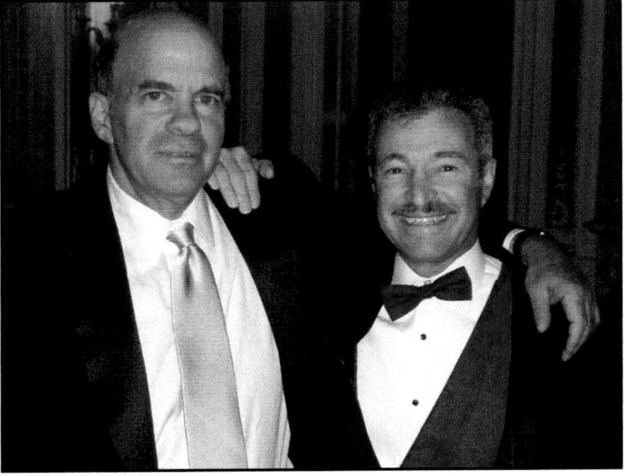

Figure 20-1. Lifelong best friend and attorney, Bob Brant.

Achievement and friendship go hand in hand. It is probably easier to achieve when there exists a network of supporting friends (Figure 20-2). For example, it is definitely easier to get back into shape when there are several individuals who share this goal and can motivate and discipline each other. My medical achievements are, in part, the result of a talented group of surgeons from around the country with whom I have been publishing and teaching for decades (Figure 20-3). Even though we do not see each other much outside of the myriad professional meetings, we always enjoy catching up whenever our paths cross, especially if we can enjoy a few laughs (Figure 20-4). I have traveled to Japan (Figure 20-5), Australia (Figure 20-6), Brazil (Figure 20-7), India (Figure 20-8), England (Figure 20-9), and Argentina when invited by good friends to a meeting that they were organizing. In my book, friends really matter!

* John Donne, *Devotions Upon Emergent Occasions—Meditation XVII*, 1624

Osher RH. *The Real ABCs: A Surgeon's Analysis and a Father's Legacy, Second Edition* (pp 95-98).

Figure 20-2. By my side deflecting 20 years of criticism, past president of the American Cataract Society, Dr. Spencer Thornton from Nashville, Tennessee.

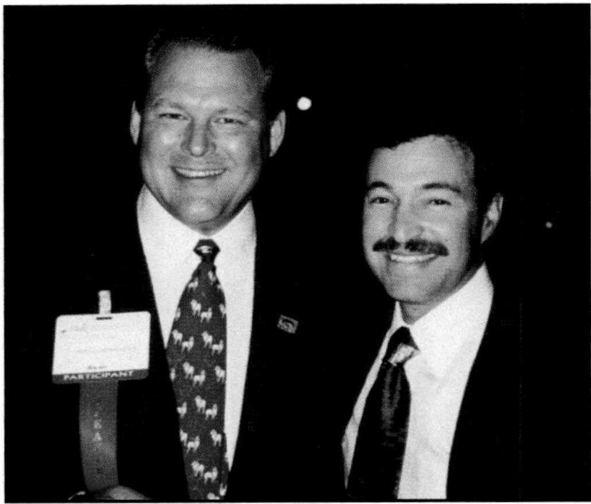

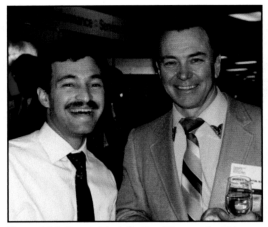

Figure 20-3. One of ophthalmology's treasures, Dr. Dick Lindstrom from Minneapolis, Minnesota and I have taught together since becoming friends in 1981.

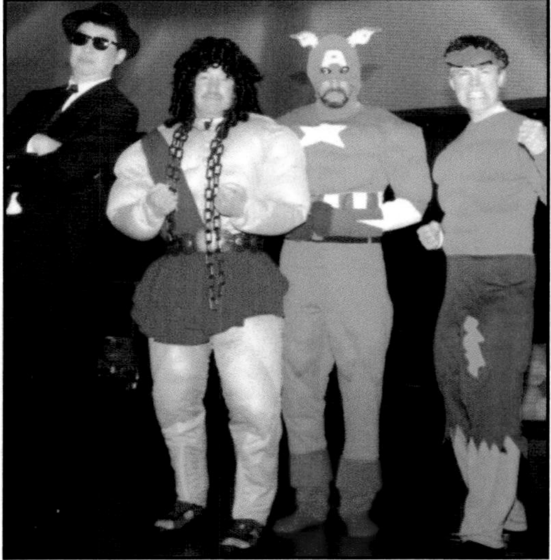

Figure 20-4. When not saving mankind, superheroes David Chang, MD; Bob Osher, MD; Dick Mackool, MD; and Doug Koch, MD are also super friends.

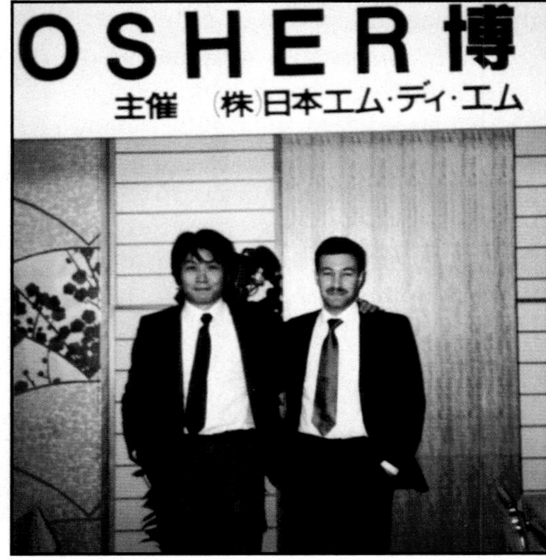

Figure 20-5. A longstanding friendship with past president of the Japanese Cataract Society, Dr. Kimiya Shimizu, makes the long trip to Tokyo worthwhile.

Another reason that Achievement and friendship go hand in hand is very important. When one achieves, it is much more satisfying to share the rewards of Achievement with friends than to bask in your glory alone. When I received the Grand Prize at the American Film Festival in 1997, it was gratifying to receive congratulatory letters and phone calls from friends around the world. When I delivered the prestigious Binkhorst Medal Lecture in 2000, awarded by the American Society of Cataract and Refractive Surgery, I was surrounded and embraced by my good friends the moment I left the podium. This makes the good times even more special.

The converse is also true. When my universe was shaken in the spring of 2003 and I was told that I had a pineapple-sized, malignant kidney tumor, I could never have arrived so quickly at a plan of action without the collaborative efforts of close friends working feverishly toward my survival. During that terrifying weekend, I had a brigade of American surgeons researching my treatment options as well as identifying the leading kidney surgeons around the country.

Figure 20-6. There is nobody I admire more than Dr. Graham Barrett, president of the Australian Cataract Society, my dear friend from Perth, Australia.

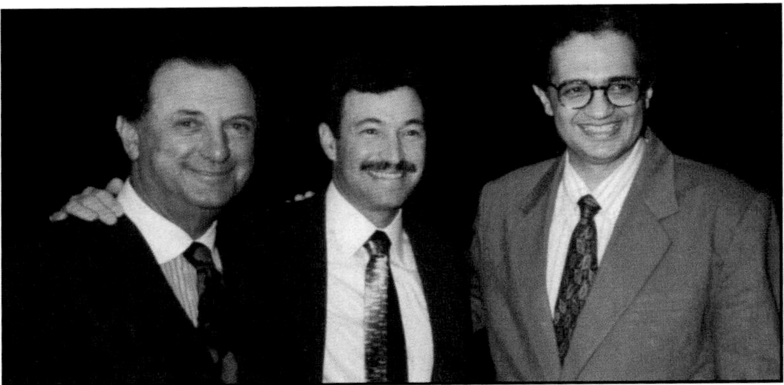

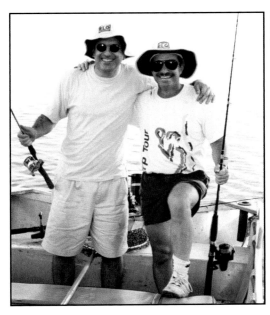

Figure 20-7. Dr. Charles Kelman, inventor of phacoemulsification, and Dr. Fernando Trindade, past president of the Brazilian Cataract Society, two friendships that I have cherished.

Figure 20-8. Renowned cataract surgeon and close friend, Dr. Abhay Vasavada, invited me to speak in India, followed by a day searching for the elusive Bengal tiger. We had to settle for a ferocious deer!

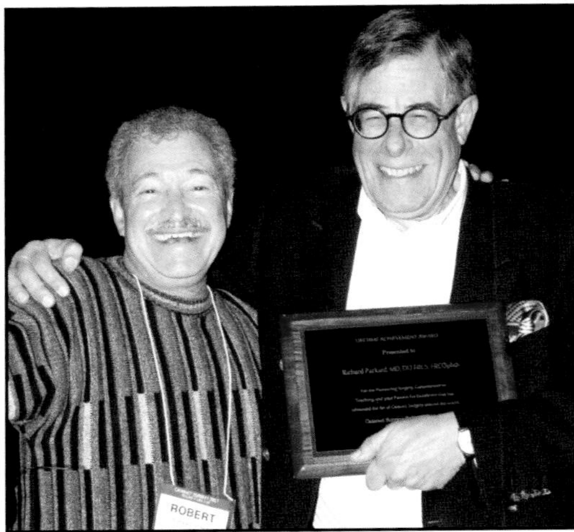

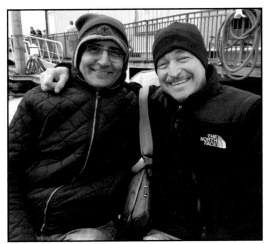

Figure 20-9. Good friend, Mr. Richard Packard, who legitimized phacoemulsification in the United Kingdom, operated on the Queen, and taught me how to fly fish.

Following my radical nephrectomy, adrenalectomy, rib removal, and extensive node dissection, the phone kept ringing with concerned voices and encouraging words of optimism. Never underestimate the power and benefit of support from friends down here and prayer up there!

As we age, our circle of good friends becomes even more cherished because we begin to realize what is really meaningful as we come to grips with our own mortality. While it is true that some of life's greatest disappointments may stem from a breach in friendship, it is also true that many of life's greatest moments are even better when shared with good friends.

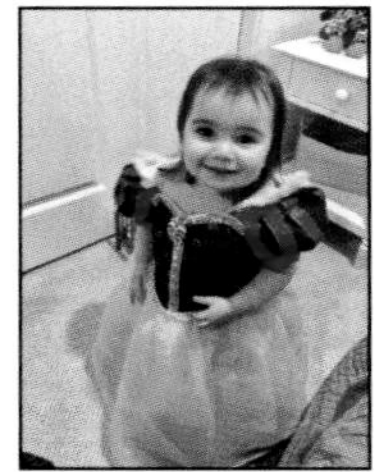

CHAPTER 21

Doing What's Right
(It's Not Always Easy)

We are each born with a conscience. Maybe it cannot be identified during an anatomic dissection of the brain, and I doubt that any radiologist has ever been able to point it out on an MRI, but it is definitely present in each of us. Granted, some people have been endowed with a very big conscience, while others could measure the size of their conscience in subatomic units. It is this ill-defined structure that accurately defines our integrity and moral constitution. While we may not know much about what makes up the conscience, perhaps more than any organ, it reveals what each of us is made of and who we are.

My parents undoubtedly tried their best to emphasize the importance of decency and moral behavior. However, with the exception of calling a close tennis shot "in" or "out," I do not recall being forced to exercise my conscience until I returned to Cincinnati, Ohio to start my practice in 1980. That is when I learned about an eye surgeon who was engaged in a Medicare scam that was clearly fraudulent. Back in those days, the surgeon received two different fees depending upon which technique he used to remove a patient's cataract. The older technique, in which the cataract was removed in one large piece (like taking an M&M* out of the eye), was reimbursed at a lower level than the newer method developed by Dr. Kelman—phacoemulsification—in which the cataract was fragmented into tiny particles by ultrasonic energy through a very small incision. If the older, large-incision technique was used, the surgeon was required by law to send the cataract to a pathologist, who would confirm that the tissue removed was nothing other than a cataract. However, if the phacoemulsification technique was used, there was no pathology specimen because the cataract was literally turned into dust-like particles collected within a bag of fluid that was then discarded.

Now, here comes the scam. This surgeon would dictate an operative note stating that he had removed the cataract by phacoemulsification, which he would then submit to Medicare for a higher payment. Yet, he was really using the older technique, and to avoid receiving the lower payment, he sent the pathology specimen to a lab across the state line. By this deceptive ploy, he received the higher payment for the older technique, and because the cataract specimen had been received in another state where the Medicare carrier was different, there was no way that this ingenious scam could be exposed. To further sweeten the pot, Medicare would pay for an extra preoperative test to assess the corneal cell count if the surgeon was performing the newer technique. The lure of easy, free money clearly seduced this surgeon who was otherwise a very likeable guy.

---

* Mars, Inc

Osher RH. *The Real ABCs: A Surgeon's Analysis and a Father's Legacy, Second Edition* (pp 99-102).

Someone in his office caught on to the scam and notified Medicare, who requested that I review his medical and financial records. As soon as I understood the fraudulent details, internal warning lights began flashing. I was trying to build a referral practice, and it is not popular to take a stand against a member of your own tribe, who in this case, was a very popular ophthalmologist. Moreover, he was from a wealthy family who would have access to the best lawyers that money could buy. Besides, I liked the guy enough to occasionally play tennis with him on Sundays.

This is where conscience comes into play. After considerable soul searching and a series of sleepless nights, I agreed to render an expert opinion stating that this behavior was dishonest. The surgeon was eventually indicted by the Federal Government. Tragically, he was a qualified surgeon whose greed led to the suspension of his medical license.

Fast forward almost 2 decades. A local news station had received so many complaints about an eye surgeon practicing in an outlying rural community that they initiated an investigation. At the request of the lead reporter, I was willing to provide a second opinion for a handful of patients who were scheduled to undergo cataract surgery. I was shocked and horrified to find that not a single patient needed the operation. These senior citizens had gone to the doctor for a routine examination, and most did not even have any symptoms. Yet, they trusted their physician when he told them that they had to have an operation to save their eyesight. My shock turned to indignation as patient after patient retold the same story. Not only was each pressured to schedule surgery, but to make matters worse, many of these same patients had already undergone multiple operations for alleged "glaucoma" performed by this same doctor. When a cataract is removed, there is no remaining evidence of whether the surgery was justified. By contrast, glaucoma causes permanent damage to the optic nerve, which is easily detected. These patients all had normal optic nerves and did not even have glaucoma!

In the first legal case, I had rendered an opinion concerning a misguided surgeon who was performing indicated surgery and then benefiting financially by a dishonest coding scam. The second situation was much worse because elderly patients were being led like sheep to slaughter, into the operating room for unnecessary surgeries. The dilemma was even more difficult because this surgeon had a group of competent partners whom I liked and respected. He was also well connected in our state political arena. When a renowned attorney filed a class action suit against this surgeon and asked for my assistance, a number of my partners strongly urged me to avoid getting involved. My conscience was unable to tolerate how he had raped the Hippocratic Oath, and I agreed to serve as the expert witness for the plaintiffs.

Nearly 3 years of intense preparation preceded the trial. Despite my pointing out the altered records and obvious inconsistencies to the jury, the surgeon managed to retain his medical license. However, the jury did render a sizable monetary verdict against him, which included several million dollars in punitive damages. Even amidst personal incriminations on the stand and serious threats that I received outside of the courtroom, I knew that I had done the right thing. Sadly, this surgeon is still practicing and scamming patients by performing unnecessary retinal and glaucoma laser procedures.

Let's look at another example. The American Society of Cataract and Refractive Surgery (ASCRS) has become the leading scientific organization dedicated to advancing cataract and refractive surgery in the United States. In its early years, however, the society lacked a disclosure policy. This meant that a surgeon who was lecturing or presenting the results of a study did not have to acknowledge that he was a paid consultant, a shareholder, or receiving a royalty from a company whose product he was discussing. This was a very dangerous omission since every member of the audience deserved to know if the speaker was financially incentivized. While I did not see anything wrong with company-sponsored research, consulting, or even royalties, I thought it was very wrong for a surgeon to promote a product for which he was being paid but fail to acknowledge this relationship.

In the mid-1980s, I wrote a strong letter to the president of the ASCRS recommending that the organization should immediately adopt a disclosure policy. I was unsatisfied with the answer that I received, so I wrote an even stronger letter to the executive committee. After receiving no response other than a verbal "back off" from the powerful program chairman, I approached members of the scientific advisory board and urged each to push for this policy, which would enhance the integrity of the society. I am quite certain that my perseverance was offensive to some of the more powerful individuals in the society, and I am equally certain that my viewpoint was in the minority. Yet, the truth is never defined by the majority opinion! Over time, the ASCRS developed the same disclosure guidelines shared by most scientific organizations. It is disappointing that my efforts were initially rebuffed, but I know that I tried to do the right thing.

I can recall another entertaining and somewhat costly incident in which my conscience played a major role. I had been invited to a lecture to a large group of eye surgeons at the Medical University of South Carolina. The meeting was held at Kiawah Island, and a golf tournament was scheduled on the famous Ocean course in the afternoon. Although it was my first year playing, I was invited to participate, and since I did not have an established handicap, an 18 was assigned to me by the organizing committee. I played in the scramble with a group of high handicappers and, because I managed to shoot 90, we found ourselves in first place. The individual prize was a $400 gift certificate at the golf shop, which I spent on unnecessary clothing. As I drove back to the hotel with one of the better golfers from the group whom had finished second, I questioned what I was supposed to do if I accidently hit a wrong ball. He explained that this error required a mandatory 2-stroke penalty which, of course, I had not realized. Nothing further was said until the next morning, when I announced to the audience from the podium that I had inadvertently "cheated" by being unaware of the 2-stroke penalty. I apologized and handed a $400 check to the meeting coordinator. Later that day, I departed from Kiawah Island with ridiculously expensive clothing, an expanded knowledge of the rules, and a clear conscience!

Another, more recent, incident comes to mind. My favorite professional club is the International Intra-Ocular Implant Club, an international group of renowned surgeons who share a history of significant contributions to the field of cataract surgery. It is a great honor to be invited to join this prestigious organization founded by the European pioneers of cataract surgery. A few years ago, an outstanding, highly opinionated surgeon who had made numerous important contributions over his 4-decade career was nominated. For inexplicable reasons, he was blackballed and denied membership. After trying to deal with my outrage from this injustice, I decided to exercise the only drastic measure that might bring attention to this travesty and result in a major overhaul of the flawed membership selection process. In other words, I resigned! In a letter that went to every member around the world, I pleaded for reform so that the founding principles of "membership based upon merit" rather than personality could be restored. I really miss being part of this group, but sometimes, it is necessary to make a personal sacrifice for a just cause.

One of my favorite movies that I have produced, which won a first prize in America and in Europe, was entitled *FDA or DWR*. This satire showed a series of international smuggling scenes in which I illegally imported sight-saving products that were unapproved by the U.S. Food and Drug Administration (FDA), and therefore, unavailable for use in the United States. At the end of the video, the audience learns that every surgeon must eventually make a difficult choice... follow FDA guidelines or DWR—Do What's Right!

Taking a moral stand can be both unpopular and uncomfortable. Still, we would be better off heeding the advice of the sage Jiminy Cricket: "Always let your conscience be your guide."

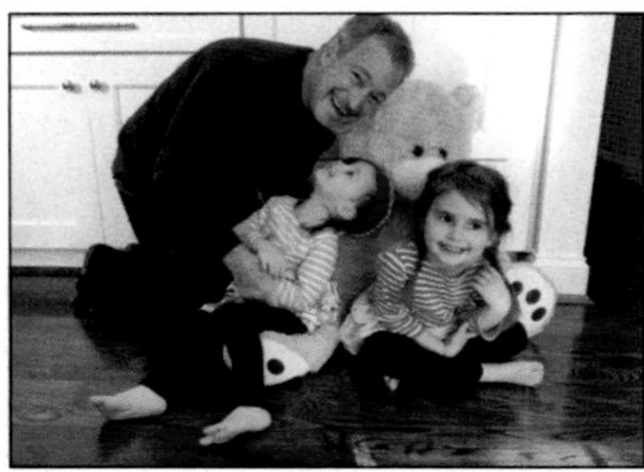

CHAPTER 22

Dream. Try. Fail. Try Harder!

Each of us is allowed to dream. As stated in an earlier chapter, wishful fancy is a good thing. Well, one of my dreams was to become an author. I had no desire to write a definitive medical textbook or a best-selling novel. Not me. I just wanted to author a series of children's stories. Why? I am not quite sure, except that I have enjoyed telling my children bedtime stories from the time they were born. Every night, I would look forward to the ritual of making up stories or composing songs on a keyboard, igniting a young imagination, or tickling a funny bone before each child drifted off to sleep. Because I was lucky enough to have five children, I have had a lot of practice telling stories. When my fifth child was about age 4, I would occasionally try to schedule my surgery starting time later in the morning so that I could visit her classroom and tell stories to the children. There is something wonderful about making a child smile, giggle, or laugh. A number of teachers had even suggested that I submit the stories for publication, but I never gave their advice much consideration.

Then, my world was turned upside down when I was diagnosed with kidney cancer. Suddenly, I had to prioritize what was really important in my life, and the stories seemed like a worthwhile legacy to leave for my children. I began writing, attempting to reconstruct characters and themes from memory, but many of my old favorites were long forgotten. With the help of my kids, I was able to recall about 20 tales, enough to advertise for an illustrator. Fortunately, a young graduate of a local art school responded, and she was both enthusiastic and talented. She was a single mother with three children under the age of 5 and desperately needed the work, so I hired her on the spot.

To my surprise, I learned that putting together a children's book is far from child's play! The paragraphs did not correlate with the illustrations, and I often wished I had paid more attention in high school English. The number of pages was not divisible by four and the illustrations' sizes and margins failed to meet the printing requirements. While I knew very little about the mechanics of publishing, I had confidence that 30 years of educating (physicians) and another 30 years of coaching (children) should somehow qualify me for the job. We managed to put together a mockup of a book about a lightning bug whose light had burned out (Figure 22-1). The first publisher to whom I sent the book offered me a contract, but only on the condition that I fire the illustrator. It would have been unconscionable to write books about values and then abandon this young artist. So, I walked away from my very first (and last) book deal. I sent out several samples to other major New York publishers and received one rejection letter after another.

Osher RH. *The Real ABCs: A Surgeon's Analysis and a Father's Legacy, Second Edition* (pp 103-109).

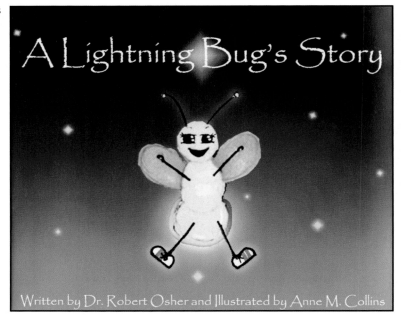

Figure 22-1. My first children's story was about a lightning bug whose light burned out before discovering the real meaning of courage.

At this point, it would have been very easy to give up. However, I have learned that rejection can actually be a very powerful incentive, and I reassured my young illustrator that we were right on course since nothing worthwhile ever came easy. My way of dealing with rejection has always been the same—I just work harder! I would not let loose of this dream and kept writing story after story.

Sometimes, when we least expect it, things have a way of working out for the best. Toward the end of the year, I was contacted by Beech Acres, a wonderful organization devoted to helping foster children, abused children, underprivileged children, etc. They were inquiring about their annual Christmas party for which I had provided gifts for decades. I mentioned to their president, Jim Mason, that I was taking a stab at writing children's books, and he offered to review them. A few days after sending him several of the mockup copies, he asked me if I would be interested in exhibiting the books at the Cincinnati Convention Center during the "For the Love of Kids" national conference. However, there was a slight timing problem because the conference was only 3 weeks away. I had absolutely no clue about how to get the books published in time to meet the deadline. Nevertheless, I accepted the challenge, found two superb local publishing companies, and had three books completed in time for a scheduled 30-minute signing during an intermission at this huge event. To my surprise, the signing lasted one-and-a-half hours and generated a lot of money, all of which I was thrilled to donate to Beech Acres.

Word of mouth traveled fast, and in the first year, I had committed to six additional book signings to raise money for other charitable organizations (Figure 22-2). Eight stories were inventoried at a local bookstore where one signing drew nearly 300 people (Figure 22-3). At last count, a total of 16 stories have been published. I know that the stories are having a positive impact on youngsters while giving parents another reason to finish the day curled up next to their little one(s). I have enjoyed reading these stories to the children at school when invited by a grandchild (Figure 22-4). Because every penny is donated to children's charities, these stories are also having a positive impact in our community. Selfishly, I am leaving my own children with a small legacy that will serve to remind them of their dad's love. I did not need the approval of a publisher to become a writer; I just needed to believe that I could do it.

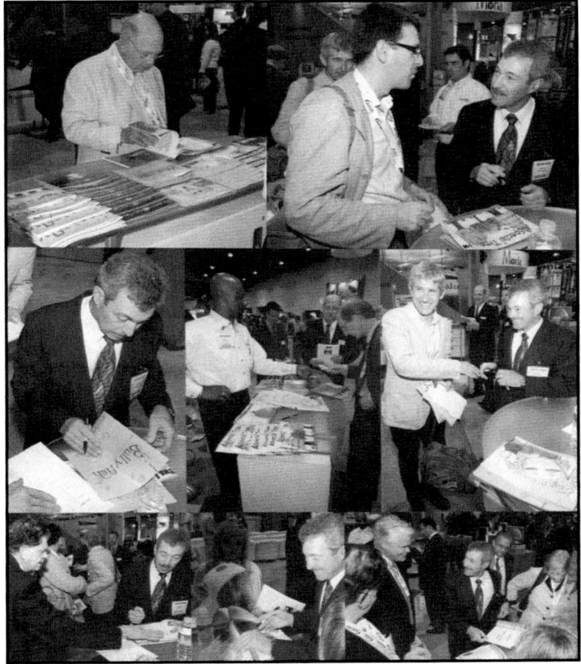

Figure 22-2. I feel privileged to be able to raise money for worthwhile organizations dedicated to helping children.

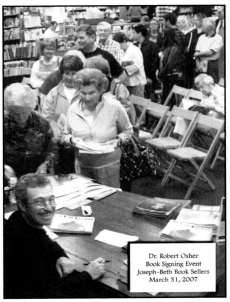

Figure 22-3. Signing books until my hand is in tetany is actually a very good feeling.

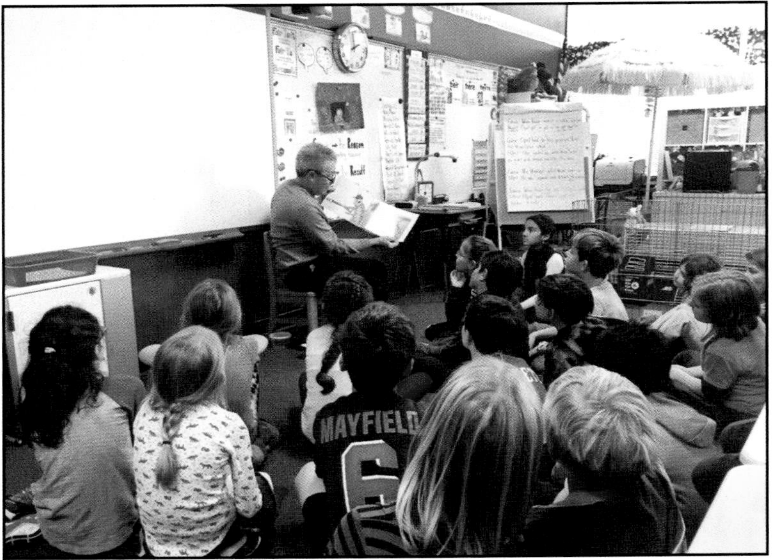

Figure 22-4. I love reading to the children at school.

While the story about writing children's books had a happy ending, I have certainly encountered my share of failures when I thought I had a good idea that flopped. In the early 1980s, I approached Ban Hudson, the president of U.S. Shoe, with the concept of a senior athletic shoe. I was beginning to experience knee pain when I was running or playing tennis, and I was convinced that there was a novel solution unknown to the shoe industry. I had been involved in the early development of ophthalmic viscoelastic devices (OVD), a protective jelly used during

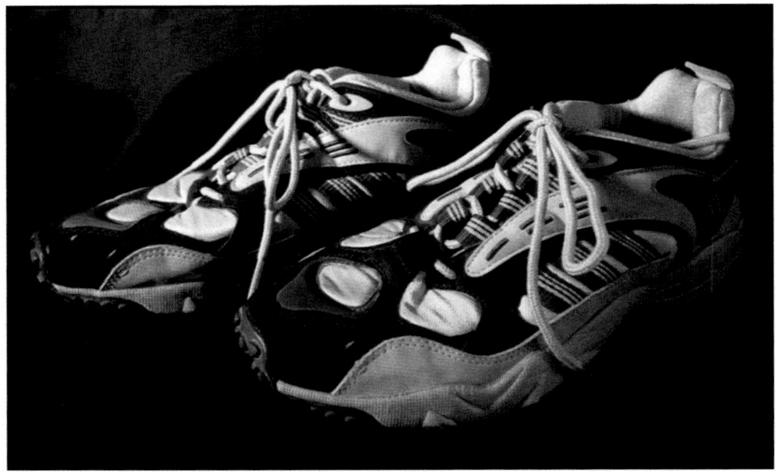

Figure 22-5. The first viscoelastic shoe for seniors.

eye surgery, and was flying back and forth to Uppsala, Sweden, to help develop the second generation of the Healon products (Johnson & Johnson). This remarkable viscoelastic agent was synthesized from rooster combs and had found an important role in cataract surgery. By lubricating the inside of the cornea, the precious endothelial cells were protected during surgery, which was a major breakthrough. A unique property of this OVD was remarkable shock absorption, and a small quantity placed on a piece of glass would prevent breakage even when heavy ball bearings were dropped onto a glass slide. I envisioned that the same amazing shock absorption could be utilized in the sole of an athletic shoe. I convinced Mr. Hudson that the recent popularity of tennis and golf tournaments specifically for seniors was the beginning of a major trend that would cater to the future baby boomers. I gave him a syringe of Healon, and he promised to discuss this idea with his research and development team.

Several weeks later, he told me that the idea had resonated well within the company, and he introduced me to a group in Colorado assigned to develop the channels that would be located in the heel of the shoe and would disperse the viscoelastic material on the strike and quickly allow it to reaccumulate. I was surprised at how fast they were able to create a model, and the shock-absorbing hypothesis was tested and confirmed. To my surprise, an executive decision was made to send the idea to Adidas, who made the first prototype (Figure 22-5).Unfortunately, the company decided that the shoe would be too expensive to manufacture, and they cancelled the project.

Disappointed but not discouraged, I contacted Philip Knight, the president of Nike, and described the idea. I was instructed to send all of my prior work to the legal department and, to make a long story short, they also declined. One of the Nike attorneys called me to explain that, although they liked the idea very much, they were going to commercialize their own new concept of using "air." Naturally, I was disappointed by the rejection, and it was frustrating to see both the success of the Nike Air line and the eventual introduction of Adidas Gel. From this experience, I learned that it might be easier to work with health care companies in the future. However, I did walk away with a free pair of shoes!

I tried taking another idea to a local health care company, Proctor & Gamble (P&G), about 5 or 10 years later. After coaching a group of youngsters in a baseball game, one of the fathers introduced himself as an executive in the health care division. I asked him if I could discuss an idea regarding dental hygiene. He seemed receptive, perhaps because I was a pretty good coach, or more likely, because P&G had just purchased the idea of a spin toothbrush from my

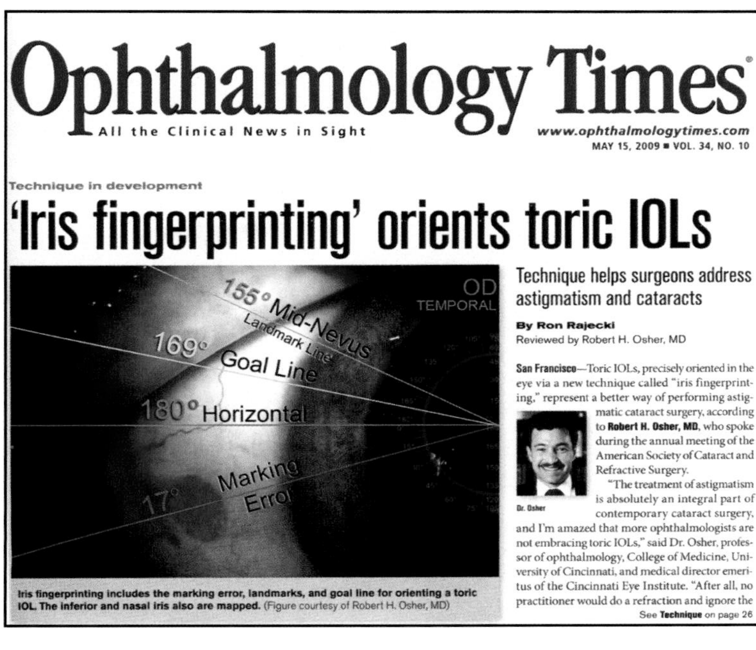

Ophthalmology Times®

All the Clinical News in Sight

www.ophthalmologytimes.com

MAY 15, 2009 ■ VOL. 34, NO. 10

Technique in development

'Iris fingerprinting' orients toric IOLs

Iris fingerprinting includes the marking error, landmarks, and goal line for orienting a toric IOL. The inferior and nasal iris also are mapped. (Figure courtesy of Robert H. Osher, MD)

Technique helps surgeons address astigmatism and cataracts

By Ron Rajecki

Reviewed by Robert H. Osher, MD

San Francisco—Toric IOLs, precisely oriented in the eye via a new technique called "iris fingerprinting," represent a better way of performing astigmatic cataract surgery, according to **Robert H. Osher, MD**, who spoke during the annual meeting of the American Society of Cataract and Refractive Surgery.

Dr. Osher

"The treatment of astigmatism is absolutely an integral part of contemporary cataract surgery, and I'm amazed that more ophthalmologists are not embracing toric IOLs," said Dr. Osher, professor of ophthalmology, College of Medicine, University of Cincinnati, and medical director emeritus of the Cincinnati Eye Institute. "After all, no practitioner would do a refraction and ignore the

See **Technique** on page 26

Figure 22-6. A new technology for using anatomic landmarks for alignment of astigmatism-correcting implants.

cousin, John Osher. Rumor has it that this little transaction was in the $200 million range. He requested that I send him a formal letter rather than introduce the idea by third base. My idea was aimed at benefiting lovers who would awaken each morning with "minty fresh breath." I suggested that a sustained-release pellet of mint could easily be attached to a tooth or the roof of the mouth at bedtime. The morning alarm goes off, and the day begins with a nice fresh kiss. Who wouldn't like that? I guess P&G didn't, because several weeks later, I was informed that there was little interest from the dental division, a decision that probably prevented millions of unplanned pregnancies!

So, I concluded that it was better to avoid working with companies specializing in shoes and health care; I resolved to stick to ophthalmology. Even within the specialty where I have a reasonably good reputation, I encountered my share of failures. For example, when astigmatism-correcting intraocular lenses were introduced, I developed an automated technology that would allow the surgeon to accurately align the toric lens for maximal astigmatism reduction. I found it quite absurd that we were removing the cataract with the most sophisticated machines, implanting highly complex intraocular lenses with advanced optics, yet the standard of care for astigmatism reduction was to use a $1.00 ink pen to place an ink mark on the sclera where the surgeon "guesstimated" the optimal orientation of the lens. Not only were these ink marks inaccurate, but they would diffuse and, in some cases, entirely disappear. My work on several sophisticated computerized technologies that would result in precise alignment of the intraocular lens did not generate much interest (Figure 22-6). Moreover, I also developed ThermoDot with Beaver-Visitec International, a method of placing a pinpoint dot(s) that would neither diffuse nor disappear in order to facilitate the accurate orientation of the lens implant (Figure 22-7). This was such an obvious solution that would improve clinical outcomes, yet the idea was never embraced by my surgical colleagues.

Another failure that I still cannot understand was the design of a new bevel-down phacoemulsification tip. Let me explain. Alcon, one of the leading companies in eye surgery, developed a new way to emulsify the cataract more efficiently using torsional ultrasound. The

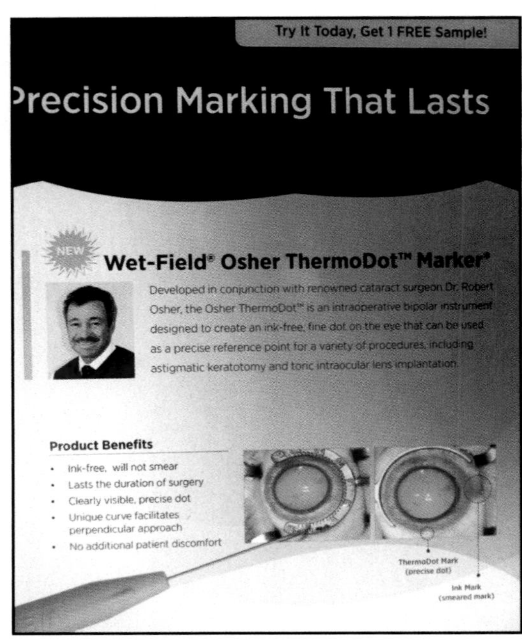

Figure 22-7. ThermoDot should replace ink, but fails.

traditional tip motion would be analogous to a jackhammer going back and forth, throwing multiple microscopic punches at the cataract. The improved torsional ultrasound would rotate back and forth, clockwise then counterclockwise, eliminating much of the punching action and improving efficiency. Historically, the tip has a bevel-up hole at the end, which has never made sense to me because it directs the ultrasonic energy up toward the cornea instead of downward toward the cataract. Moreover, when the hole is up, it tends to break up and remove the protective jelly (OVD) mentioned earlier in this chapter. My idea was to reverse the tip bevel so the hole would be facing downward, directing the energy into the cataract and leaving the protective OVD undisturbed. Alcon developed the prototypes, which worked extremely well, directing the energy backward through the first half of the cataract while allowing the OVD to provide exquisite protection to the cornea that did not even “know” I was working. Then, after removing some of the cataract and cracking it into pieces, I would rotate the tip upward to avoid encountering the fragile capsular membrane in the back of the cataract. It worked great, so I sent several samples to other leading surgeons, who were very impressed. Unfortunately, Alcon canceled the rollout, and although the tip is still available, the company chose to go in a different direction. I continue to use this tip in all of my cases, as does the busiest surgeon in Japan, but I think we may constitute a minority of two (Figure 22-8)!

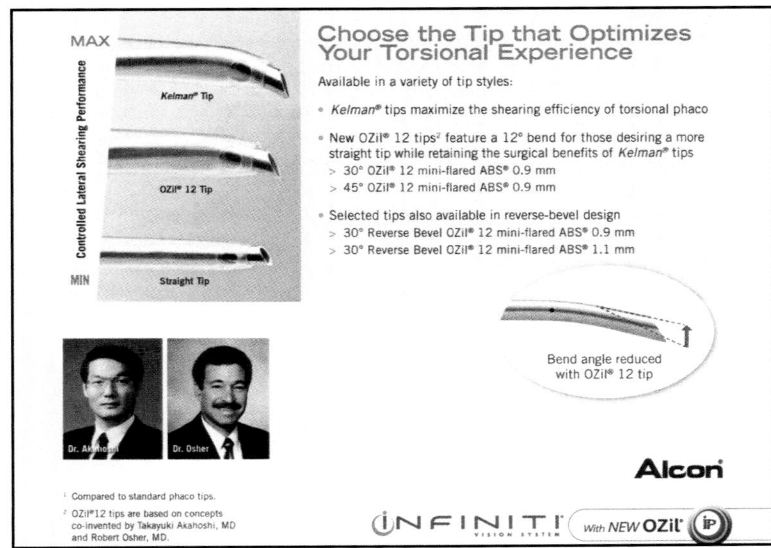

Figure 22-8. New bevel-down phacoemulsification tip goes belly-up.

Throughout history, ideas and accomplishments are usually rejected and criticized long before becoming accepted. This pattern is quite predictable and represents basic human nature. So, expect rejection, refuse to take it personally, believe in yourself, and be willing to persevere until the goal is reached. If things do not work out, at least you tried. If you do not try, things will never work out. Remember, the steep uphill road gives the best view from the top!

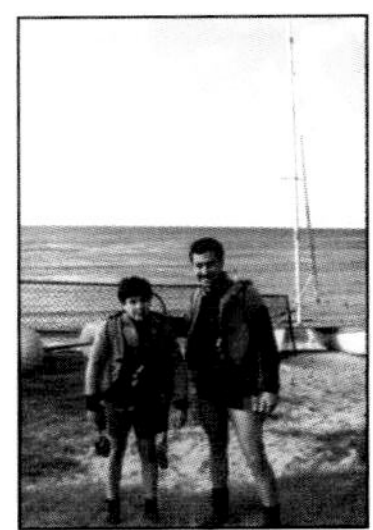

CHAPTER 23

Dealing With Adversity

Bad things always happen to somebody else, the other guy, about whom we read in the newspaper. Wrong! I always thought that I was virtually indestructible. Wrong! How about living on planet Earth forever? Wrong again. Sooner or later, each of us is going to encounter adversity or a catastrophic event that really changes our lives. For me, it was sooner.

When I reached my mid-50s, I decided to take up golf, primarily for social reasons. Between lectures that I delivered to the Canadian Masters Society Winter Meeting in Tucson, Arizona, I snuck away to play a beautiful course nestled in the mountains. On the 16th tee, I experienced some tingling down my right leg. Having had a neurology background, I suspected that this symptom represented some mild lower back strain arising from too many golf swings, and I did not think much about it. The following day, when I returned to Cincinnati, Ohio, I was walking to my office through the parking lot and happened to run into a friend of mine who practices neurology. He asked why I was limping, and he encouraged me to have an MRI scan. It is unusual for me to have 1 hour free and even more unusual when I follow someone's advice on such short notice. The MRI team had an opening, so I had a quick scan of my back. The following morning, the phone rang, and the radiologist began by saying that I was right about the mild disc irritation, which he added was the "good news." He continued by informing me of the bad news…the scan showed a pineapple-sized, malignant kidney tumor! My first response was to ask whose name was on the MRI report since it could not possibly be mine. It was.

Within moments, my entire universe collapsed and crumbled. Almost paralyzed with fear, I returned that afternoon for additional MRI tests, which reconfirmed this terrible diagnosis (Figure 23-1). A suffocating helplessness set in, and I was overwhelmed with thoughts of my 6-year-old daughter. Who would clean her glasses? Who would protect her? Who would teach her how to catch (Figure 23-2)?

During the next 2 days, I called dozens of my colleagues around the country, asking for their urgent help in contacting the top experts in kidney cancer at their respective universities. My friends responded, and my cell phone rang continuously as America's most prestigious renal oncologists called with their recommendations for saving my life. From my own personal experience, I knew that I needed a pure subspecialist with years of experience in order to maximize my chances for survival. While the common consensus was a physician at the Cleveland Clinic, there was considerable debate regarding the small- versus large-incision approach. I had heard this debate many times in cataract surgery, and the small-incision approach was clearly the superior eye operation. However, my brother, Sandy, a gynecology specialist, convinced me that the goal was not faster rehabilitation nor a small scar. He believed that filleting me wide open

Osher RH. *The Real ABCs: A Surgeon's Analysis and a Father's Legacy, Second Edition* (pp 111-113).

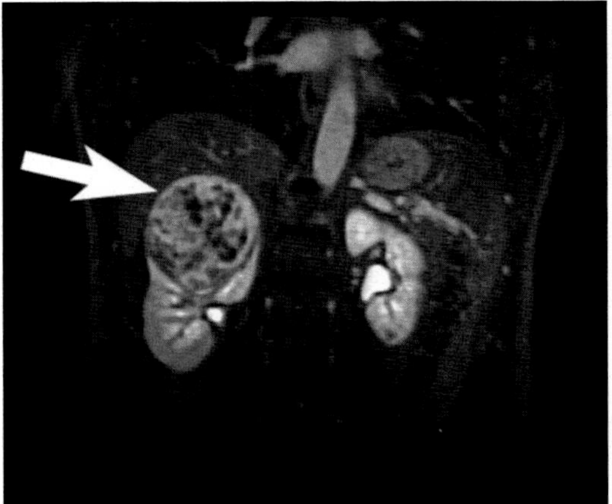

Figure 23-1. The MRI showed a pineapple-sized, malignant kidney tumor.

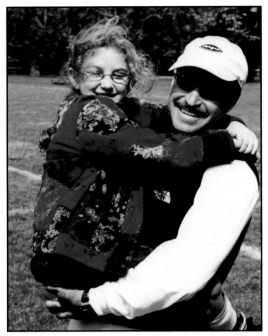

Figure 23-2. I could not just die. Jessie needed someone to clean her glasses.

would give the surgeon the best possible visualization of the cancer with less risk of leaving malignant tumor behind.

On Sunday evening, after completing 48 hours of intensive research, I called my children together in our living room. Looking at their beautiful faces and knowing that I might not see them again was the most excruciatingly painful experience ever. On Monday, I performed six operations and then drove to the Cleveland Clinic, where the MRI was to be repeated. I sunk into the depths of depression as I sat waiting for my turn, observing the young children who were also undergoing testing for their fatal cancers. I had already led a very full life, and it did not seem fair that these little ones may never be given the opportunity to do so.

Several hours later, I met my surgeon, Andrew Novick, MD, the Chairman of the Department of Urology and a world-renowned expert in renal cell cancer. I appreciated his candor and felt confident in his hands. The arrival of my wife and sister was reassuring, yet it also underscored that the diagnosis and operation were very serious. We were informed that there was a possibility that the procedure could take 4 hours and that I might not awaken. I wrote letters to each of my children professing my love, while expressing my belief that, even in death, I would always be a source of their strength. The minister came in and asked us all to hold hands as he recited the Lord's Prayer. At that moment, I reminded my family that the last time a group of us held hands and recited the Lord's Prayer, my basketball team had been beaten by 20 points! Hopefully, I would do better this time around. I was wheeled into the cold operating room. I smiled at the scrub nurse and reminded her that it was my RIGHT kidney. I closed my eyes, folded my arms across my chest, addressed my creator, and felt surprisingly comfortable and at peace.

When I awoke, I was immediately aware of tubes and hoses in every possible orifice. Next, I noted a profound inability to move my body without an indescribable searing pain, but I was alive! I have a vague recollection of a discussion during which the surgeon told me he had removed a rib, the kidney, the adrenal gland, and all of the nodes along the aorta. He reassured me that the surgery had gone well, in part because I was in excellent physical shape. Perhaps, I had just imagined this comment since I was not in good enough shape to even sit up in bed. Within 24 hours, I was forcing myself to walk, and 1 or 2 days later, I was jogging laps while pushing my intravenous pole through the hospital corridors, much to my nurse's dismay! One week later, I was discharged, and I tackled a full operating room schedule the following Monday. That afternoon, I forced myself to chip a bucket of golf balls around the green. My cell phone rang, and a physician explained the pathology report, which indicated that the cancer was highly malignant, but there was no evidence of metastatic spread elsewhere. I felt optimistic and knocked a 15-yard chip off the pin into the cup.

During the next several months, I worked hard to regain my strength and fitness. Yet, the most remarkable part of my recovery was mental rather than physical. I experienced an enormous transformation in my attitude and a new appreciation for practically everything. A simple conversation with my children was precious. My relationship with my wife, which had varied somewhere between stormy and disastrous, markedly improved. Realizing she had been by my side, I tried to re-energize a failing marriage. The many small problems at work, which used to drive me crazy, no longer seemed to matter. In fact, I was grateful just to be around to try to solve them. Nature's smallest gifts, which previously went unnoticed, were treasured. The splendor of a butterfly's color and the magnificence of a simple sunset made me feel euphoric. Not a minute was wasted as I attempted to "seize every moment." Within 2 months, I was back to coaching, jogging, and tossing in the kayak for a run down the river. My work became even more rewarding, my friendships became more meaningful, and my life was never so good.

There are several ways to deal with adversity, and I chose the approach where every moment of every day is a gift and a blessing. As a result, I was living my life more fully than ever before. Long after midnight in the early morning hours, I do not fall asleep before giving thanks that yesterday was a near perfect day. I close my eyes believing that when I awaken in a few hours, today will be even better. And with respect to tomorrow, if need be, I'll worry about tomorrow, tomorrow.

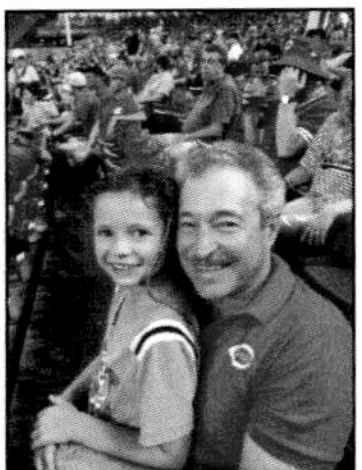

CHAPTER 24

Resilience

We often use words like *integrity*, *courage*, *wisdom*, and *kindness* when expressing admiration for human behavior. Not very often does the word *resilience* come to mind. Yet, the ability to recover from the setbacks that every living creature encounters may define a city, team, or individual. When things go wrong, typical reactions may include anger, sadness, frustration, self-pity, despair, or even "tossing in the towel" and giving up. However, the trait of resilience is an ingredient so important that success rarely comes without it. A perfect example of resilience is the fictional character, Rocky Balboa, the Italian Stallion from the streets of Philly. Audiences fell in love with his gritty resilience as he picked himself up off the canvas time after time to overcome all odds in his pursuit of becoming the heavyweight boxing champion of the world. Real life examples include the resilience of Boston Red Sox Hall of Famer, Kevin Youkilis, who was cut from his high school baseball team, and Chicago Bulls star, Michael Jordan, who I am told encountered a similar basketball setback. The indomitable American spirit following the horrific 9/11 tragedy showed our resilience to the world, and the Boston Strong mentality following the Boston Marathon bombing would also certainly qualify.

Resilience can exist on a much smaller scale and may have helped me through a very difficult time in my life. When I was a young surgeon in the early 1980s, I received several wonderful invitations to speak at prestigious meetings. Usually, it is difficult for a youngster to get invited to speak before a national or international audience, but I had just designed an intraocular lens that had attracted considerable attention. The Annual Meeting of the American Academy of Ophthalmology was held in Chicago, Illinois in about 1983, and I received my first major invitation to speak on the subject of the torn posterior capsule, one of the most common complications at the time of cataract surgery. The capsule is the thin, cellophane-like envelope surrounding the natural lens that does the focusing for the eye. When the lens becomes cloudy, it becomes a cataract. If the fragile capsular sac (bag) located behind the iris is torn during cataract surgery, it was the standard of care to place the intraocular lens in front of the iris in a space called the *anterior chamber* near the front of the eye. It was considered too dangerous to put the lens inside the torn capsular sac. However, I did not like the anterior chamber lens, which would distort or ovalize the pupil and had other side effects like causing UGH syndrome, which stands for uveitis (inflammation), glaucoma (elevated pressure), and hyphema (bleeding inside the eye). I wanted to put the intraocular lens behind the iris into the capsular bag, the same tiny sac that held the God-given natural lens, where it was suspended in the eye away from all delicate tissues. I had done my homework, going to the operating room at night, and deliberately tearing the capsular bag in cadaver eyes. To my surprise, when I placed the intraocular lens into

Osher RH. *The Real ABCs: A Surgeon's Analysis and a Father's Legacy, Second Edition* (pp 115-118).

this torn sac, the artificial lens did not fall with gravity and disappear (as expected) into the depths of the eye. It stayed in place, bridging the central tear that I had created in the very thin (3 or 4 μm) capsule. It was amazing to observe, and it gave me the confidence to deal with this complication in a fresh, new way, resulting in a better surgical outcome. However, when I stood before thousands of eye surgeons and reported my findings, there wasn't a single applause in the audience. I was called "dangerous" and "crazy" by opinion leaders. In fact, I was not invited back to speak at the American Academy of Ophthalmology for 10 years! As a young surgeon who wanted to contribute, the pain of rejection by colleagues was overwhelming. It took many unpopular presentations over a decade, but eventually, colleagues began to place the lens behind the iris into the torn capsular bag with superior results. Resilience paid off, but my reputation was off to a shaky start.

Perhaps an even better example of resilience goes back to 1980. During my training at the number-one ranked Bascom Palmer Eye Institute in Miami, Florida, I was enthusiastic about almost everything in ophthalmology and showed a strong attraction to anything that was new in the field of ophthalmic surgery. I heard a presentation from Russian pioneer, Dr. Svyatoslav Fyodorov, about radial keratotomy, a new operation in which a series of incisions were placed on the cornea, resulting in the reduction or elimination of myopia (nearsightedness). I spent hours in the animal lab, where I began placing incisions on rabbit corneas with fragments of a carbon shaving blade. The academic establishment thought that this operation was one step from insanity, so I had to conduct my animal research secretly. When I asked permission to visit the surgeon in Deland, Florida who was one of the first to perform this operation in the United States, I was prohibited by the Chairman of the Department. So, I decided to go anyway using my limited vacation time, analyzed all of his patients, and submitted my findings to every journal in America. The manuscript was rejected by all, and I eventually had to publish this article in *Documenta Ophthalmologica* in the European literature several years later.

At around this time, I heard a brilliant ophthalmologist from Nashville, Tennessee, Dr. Spencer Thornton, discussing how incisions placed strategically on the cornea could also reduce astigmatism, which is warpage of the cornea. I hopped on a plane to visit the office of Dr. George Tate, a surgeon in Pinehurst, North Carolina, who was correcting residual high astigmatism following corneal transplantation with these corneal incisions. It struck me with the force of a tsunami: why not combine these incisions with routine cataract surgery for the reduction of *pre-existing* astigmatism!

Cataract surgeons had paid a tremendous amount of attention to reducing nearsightedness and farsightedness with the intraocular lens. There had also been a significant amount of work aimed at avoiding the creation of new astigmatism following cataract surgery. Yet, absolutely nobody was thinking about the reduction of pre-existing astigmatism in order to achieve clear vision without glasses in patients who were scheduled to undergo cataract surgery. In 1983, I began investigating the possibility of placing a very peripheral corneal incision to reduce the astigmatism and, after a second corneal incision was added, the results were dramatic. Patients with lots of astigmatism who had never been able to see well without glasses before developing their cataract were suddenly able to see clearly with unaided vision following a combined small-incision cataract procedure (phacoemulsification) with astigmatic keratotomy (corneal incisions).

I received an invitation to present this study at the Cataract Congress, which attracted more than 1000 surgeons to Houston, Texas. The unique format required that each speaker had to address a panel of nine international experts who would be free to comment on and criticize the presentation. I had collected and analyzed the results of operating upon 128 eyes, and my presentation was flawless. As my last slide dropped, I concluded that astigmatic keratotomy combined with phacoemulsification was a new, powerful, and effective way of achieving unaided vision by reducing pre-existing astigmatism. I smiled triumphantly at the panel and waited for the applause from the audience. Once again, there was none. The silence was deafening.

What followed, to put it mildly, was a bloodbath—a medical massacre! The renowned Dr. Normal Jaffe, who was the pioneer who helped to get the intraocular lens approved in the United States, began by stating that, as one of my teachers, he was appalled by my wanton disrespect for the cornea. Dr. Jan Worst, a famous eye surgeon from the Netherlands, quickly followed by stating that the cornea was the only tissue in the body that remained virgin until I had mutilated it with a knife. Those were two of the nicer comments. I remember leaving the stage feeling pommeled and embarrassed. Fortunately, I encountered a handful of people who consoled and encouraged me. The first was Charles Kelman, MD, the Father of Phacoemulsification, who put his hand on my shoulder and told me to keep my head up. He went on to say that he had been "beaten to a pulp" on many occasions, and I needed to "toughen up" and ignore the harsh criticism. Spencer Thornton, MD, the charismatic astigmatism expert, went out of his way to compliment me for introducing the idea and for completing the clinical study that seemed to justify this combined procedure. Two of my friends, Richard Lindstrom, MD, and Douglas Koch, MD, both who eventually rose to international fame, embraced this new idea of refractive cataract surgery. These four ophthalmologists gave me the collective support that I needed to become resilient. I persevered and published this new approach, which years later became accepted as a standard way to reduce astigmatism at the time of cataract surgery. Not long after, in 1985, I introduced and published another refractive procedure in which the clear natural lens of the eye was removed to correct pre-existing farsightedness. Again, I was ridiculed by outspoken critics who called me negligent, and it took decades for the criticism to finally cease. Today, clear lensectomy is an accepted option for treating farsightedness (hyperopia).

I want to close by sharing my favorite example of resilience by introducing Lucy, the tiny Yorkshire puppy that my youngest daughter, Jessica, gave to her mother. During an overnight stay at the kennel, Lucy's right front leg was tragically caught in the cage and required an emergency amputation. Picking Lucy up from the veterinary hospital several days later was one of the saddest days of my life (Figure 24-1). Yet, over time, Lucy learned to get around on three legs, and it was not long before she was dashing across the yard like any four-legged dog. Then, an incredible thing happened: she learned to sit upright (Figure 24-2) and then to walk, balanced on two legs like a human. What an amazing sight to see this little dog out for a walk… walking (Figure 24-3)! Lucy, you are my hero!

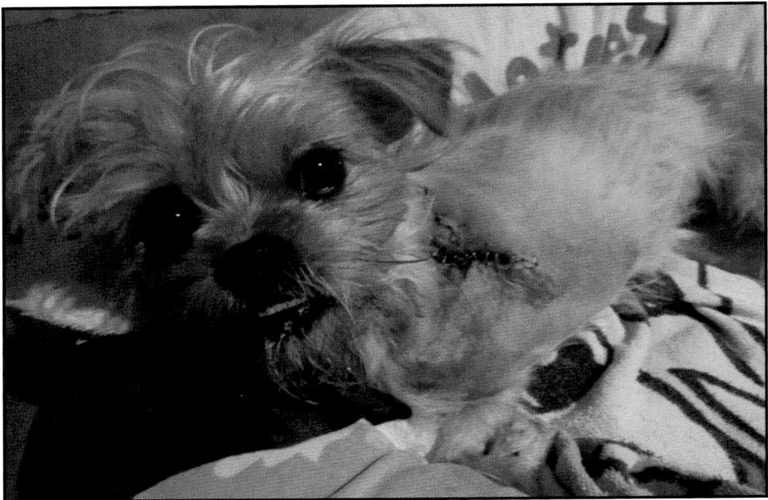

Figure 24-1. Lucy's leg was amputated…

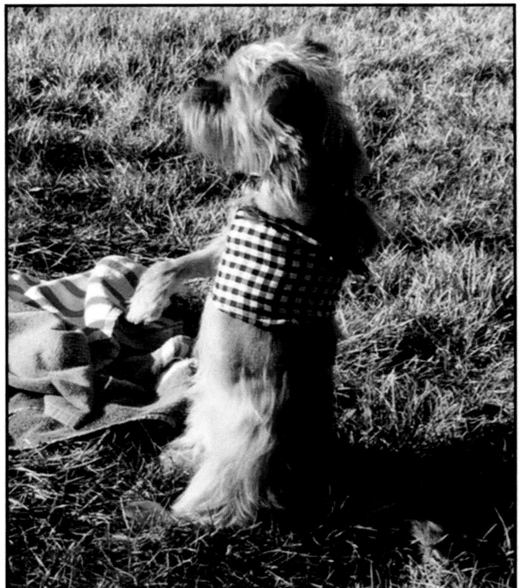

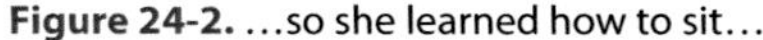

Figure 24-2. ...so she learned how to sit...

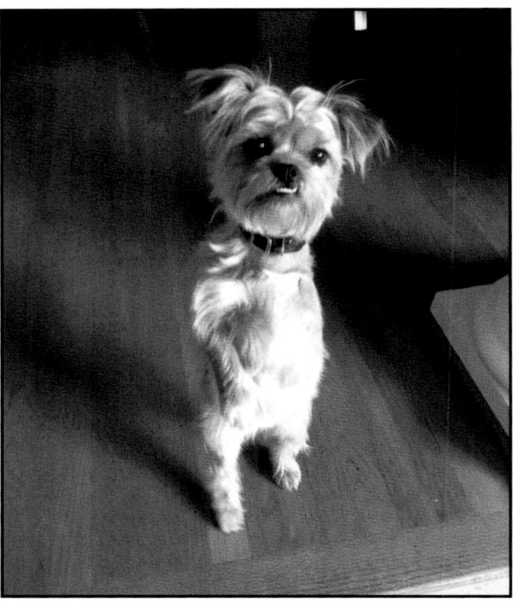

Figure 24-3. ...and then started to walk on two legs like a person.

Every person who is striving for excellence or attempting to reach a goal is going to encounter setbacks. We must expect adversity, accept adversity, and use adversity as motivation to continue the quest. Resilience is an asset, much like owning Boardwalk in the game of Monopoly*; the longer you stay in the game, the greater the chance that good things will eventually happen. If you are not familiar with Monopoly, another analogy also applies: Resilience is the appliance that transforms a lemon into lemonade.

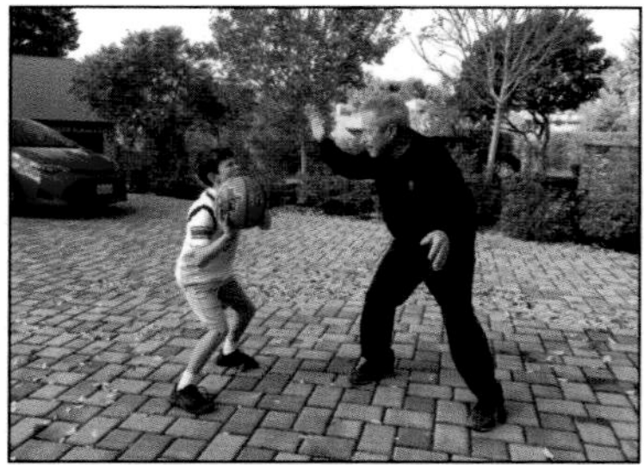

* Hasbro

CHAPTER 25

Values and Meaning

Over a lifetime, it is possible to achieve a great deal of material wealth, power, and greatness without having character or integrity. History is full of individuals with lofty accomplishments who were ruthless and amoral. Values and the way we conduct our lives are the result of the personal belief system that each of us has adopted. This belief system provides an explanation or rationale for our very existence, which, in turn, gives our lives meaning and significance.

It is virtually impossible to move along our career path with integrity unless we accept accountability for our decisions and actions. When we have faith that there is an ultimate purpose or plan for our lives, it becomes so much easier to believe in right and wrong. The game of life and the game of golf share absolute, non-negotiable rules. When I began playing golf, I was shocked when players of every caliber would move the ball to improve their lie or would quickly pick up a 4-foot putt as a "gimme." The rules of golf forbid this behavior, and it is simply unacceptable. Those who hold the game in the highest regard and assume the responsibility of their own behavior will hit the ball as it lies and will putt until the ball is resting in the bottom of the cup. It is the accountability of behavior and the respect for the "big picture" that differentiates these two groups of players.

As a physician, I hold certain truths as incontrovertible facts. Every life is precious, and every human being deserves respect until proven otherwise. Every patient should be given my best effort and should be treated as if he or she were a member of my family. I wish that every patient could be cured, but those who cannot should always be comforted.

Throughout medical school, I became increasingly impressed by the miracle of life. With the birth of each of my five children, I abandoned prior scientific training and embraced the belief that each of these miracles was neither just a melding of chromosomes nor the result of some ill-defined evolutionary process. While I do not profess an expertise in theology or religion, I acquired a profound faith that each of us is put on the Earth for a reason and given the opportunity to make a difference. While the reason and the opportunity may vary from person to person, my simple philosophy is that our lifetime should be productive, enjoyable, and played between those boundaries defined by our values. When we inevitably stray off base, we must try to get back on track. I am guilty of stumbling in my marriage, my child rearing, and in my insensitivity to those less fortunate and to the health of our planet. More than once, I have tried to reset my moral compass and aspire to be a better, more thoughtful person. Human beings err, and we must feel compelled to make things right. As in golf, there are penalties and triumphs along the way. Yet, eventually, a final score is tallied, and this what matters.

Osher RH. *The Real ABCs: A Surgeon's Analysis and a Father's Legacy, Second Edition* (pp 119-120).

The gift of life is finite, and there is never enough time to do and enjoy everything. However, when there is purpose in our lives, it is much easier to prioritize our goals, to keep them in clear focus, and to pursue them with integrity.

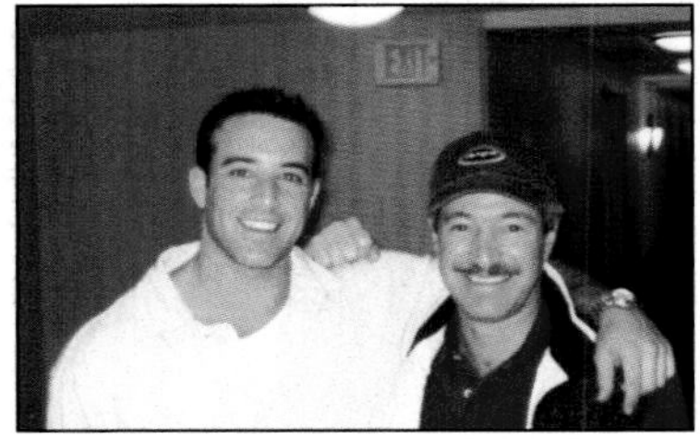

CHAPTER 26

Why I Love My Job!

As a youngster, there were only two things that I wanted to be when I grew up. My number one choice was to be a professional basketball player, but a deficiency in growth hormone convinced me to settle for my second choice, being an ophthalmologist like my father. In retrospect, it should have been my first choice because I feel like I have hit the lottery most every day. It is hard to describe the feeling of satisfaction that I get whenever I remove a cataract and help someone recover clear vision. Even though I do this day in and day out, it never gets old. Let me give you just one example.

About 10 years ago, on a Wednesday, which is my new patient clinic, I watched my devoted assistant, Dee, escort the next patient into the exam room. He was a 44-year-old man with an intellectual disability who was accompanied by each of his parents. His father had his right arm and his mother was holding his left arm as they guided him through the door and helped him into the examination chair. He had been born with congenital cataracts and was legally blind. His parents refused to institutionalize their son and had provided home care for his entire life. It was obvious that his vision was very poor because he did not acknowledge my presence as I sat down next to him. When I spoke to him, his communication skills were limited, but he was able to nod his head "yes" or "no."

My examination immediately revealed a totally white cataract in each eye, which explained the fact that he could not even see my hand waving a few inches in front of his face. It was as if he had two white snowballs, each about the size of a large M&M,* just behind the pupil, preventing any light from reaching the retina (Figure 26-1). From experience, I knew that this cataract would have a very hard center, which we affectionately call a *catarock* because it is much more difficult to remove without complications. To add to the challenge, there was no chance that he could cooperate enough to remain still for the 20-minute procedure usually performed with the patient wide awake.

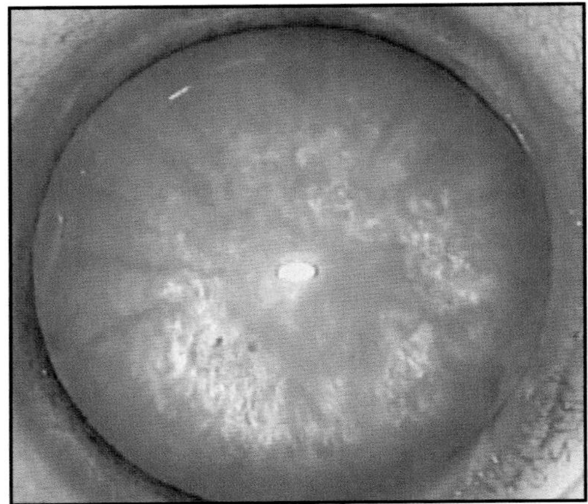

Figure 26-1. One of my patient's totally white cataracts.

* Mars, Inc

Osher RH. *The Real ABCs: A Surgeon's Analysis and a Father's Legacy, Second Edition* (pp 121-122).

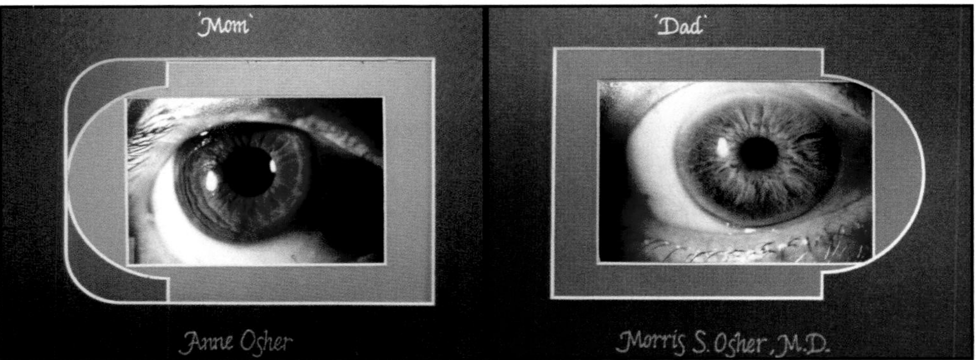

Figure 26-2. How satisfying to be able to give my parents back their sight after removing cataracts from each.

After spending considerable time explaining the operation and the highly guarded prognosis to his parents, we scheduled his surgery under general anesthesia. I had not operated under general anesthesia for at least 30 years, which added one more risk to the equation. On the day of surgery, I was very well prepared. As expected, the surgery was challenging, but I was able to remove the 10-mm cataract through a 2.2-mm incision and implant an intraocular lens. Sutures are usually unnecessary with these very small incisions, but I took an extra precaution and covered the incision with a glue-like adhesive in case the patient were to rub or bump his eye following surgery.

I always see my patients on the day following surgery, and I felt unusually nervous as I approached the exam room where he and his parents were waiting. My anxiety was heightened as I opened the door and I saw each of his parents sobbing. My first thought was that he was no better and still blind. Had the operation failed? The mother had her arms around her son and his hands were moving slowly across her cheeks. Before I could speak, she looked at me and she said, "Dr. Osher, this is the first time that my son has ever seen my face." As these words sunk in, it was not long before I was also in tears. No game-winning shot at the buzzer in front of 20,000 fans could have matched the joy that I felt at that moment.

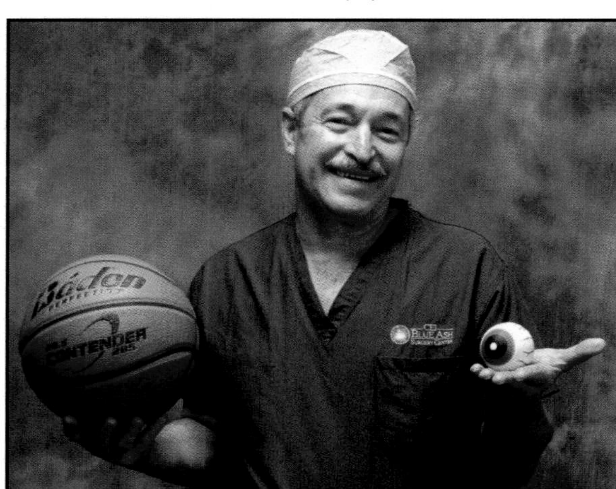

Figure 26-3. I made the right choice!

How lucky can one man get? I am not referring to this patient. I feel grateful that every day I get to do what I really enjoy, something that really makes a difference. You can't imagine the joy I felt when I was able to remove my mother's and father's cataracts (Figure 26-2). No offense to Michael Jordan or LeBron James, but I will choose eyeballs over basketballs any day of the week (Figure 26-3)!

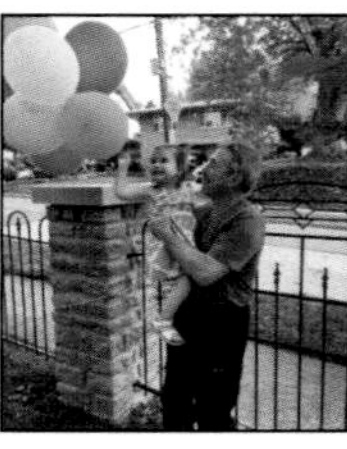

CHAPTER 27

Taking a Stand

Throughout my adult life, I have shied away from attention outside of my teaching efforts in ophthalmology. This might seem somewhat inconsistent because I am frequently in front of large groups of people, but given the choice, I would opt every time for the peace and quiet of solitude. Perhaps that is why I enjoy biking, kayaking, exercising, and even playing golf in the evening by myself. In fact, 1 year ago, I turned down an invitation to serve as the Guest of Honor at the annual philanthropic event organized by the Cincinnati Eye Institute Foundation. I really did not want to be the center of attention, which was quite a surprise to the nominating committee. More recently, I declined an invitation to have an annual lectureship bearing my name at the University of Cincinnati. This also came as a surprise, even to my own children.

However, we each must "stand up and be counted" when truly important issues arise. Maintaining the high quality of cataract surgery in the United States is extremely important to me, which explains why I accepted an invitation from the American Academy of Ophthalmology to serve as a "poster child" for the Surgical Scope Fund. This battle to safeguard millions of patients undergoing eye surgery is the result of our misguided federal and state regulatory agencies who have been led to believe that everyone should have a chance to practice medicine. How absurd!

When I went to medical school, only a qualified obstetrician could deliver babies. Today, it is done by just about anybody, even taxi drivers! When a delivery goes smoothly, everybody is happy, but if there is anything unusual (eg, my oldest daughter's vital signs ceased, necessitating an emergency C-section), then it is absolutely necessary to have a physician with the best training managing the situation.

There has been recent legislation proposed in several states that would allow non-ophthalmologists to perform eye operations, including cataract surgery. This policy might save health care dollars, but it is fraught with extreme danger. Again, if all goes well, everyone would be happy, but cataract surgery is a very difficult operation, and the patient's sight is at stake. When a complication occurs, the eye could be lost, leaving the patient blind. That is where the line should be drawn, and only a highly qualified ophthalmologist should be performing cataract surgery. To legislate surgical privileges to perform surgery inside of the eye will result in catastrophic complications, and patients will suffer.

For this reason, I have approved the following full-page ad from the American Academy of Ophthalmology, which is intended to protect patients undergoing eye surgery (Figure 27-1).

Osher RH. *The Real ABCs: A Surgeon's Analysis and a Father's Legacy, Second Edition* (pp 123-124).

Figure 27-1. I feel passionate about protecting the Gift of Sight.

STATE ADVOCACY

AMERICAN ACADEMY OF OPHTHALMOLOGY®

I believe in high surgical standards. I protect sight.

I support the Surgical Scope Fund.

"Cataract surgery is a beautiful, elegant procedure. I've spent countless hours studying, practicing, and traveling to become the best cataract surgeon I can be. It's frightening to think that this demanding procedure or any other eye surgery could be performed by anyone other than a highly-trained ophthalmic surgeon. We each took an oath to protect our patients. That's why I contribute to the Surgical Scope Fund and that's why I'm urging you to do the same."

ROBERT H. OSHER, MD
Professor of Ophthalmology, College of Medicine, University of Cincinnati; Medical Director Emeritus of Cincinnati Eye Institute

When high surgical standards are threatened nationwide, the Academy's Surgical Scope Fund can deliver resources, expertise and winning strategies for protecting patient safety and preserving surgery by surgeons.

Make your confidential Surgical Scope Fund contribution today at aao.org/ssf.

Protecting Sight. Empowering Lives.®

After 40 years of learning and teaching cataract surgery, I feel compelled to take a public stand and state that cataract surgery and other difficult ocular procedures that require a great deal of surgical training should be performed only by qualified and board-certified ophthalmic surgeons. As my quotation states, we took an oath in medical school to protect patients, and if we do not, no one else will.

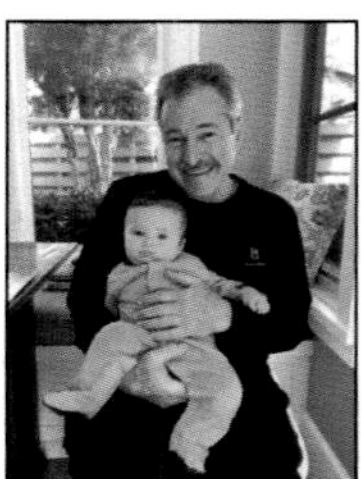

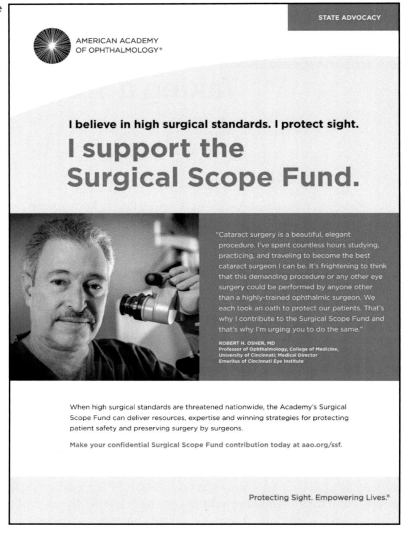

CHAPTER 28

Miracles Never Cease!

Day after day, year after year, I am continuously amazed at how many miracles, both large and small, we take for granted. As mentioned in a previous chapter, childbirth is definitely a miracle. Vision is a miracle. The human body is a miracle. Never let anyone diminish the power of self will and intense prayer. Miracles do happen! Here is a real example.

Years ago, I had just finished 1 week of lecturing and playing in a golf tournament in Kiawah Island in South Carolina, and my lower back was really sore (sound familiar?). The symptoms steadily worsened until I had severe, constant pain radiating down each leg. After an MRI scan, two different world-class radiologists looked at the films and exclaimed, "Wow, you have a huge extruded lumbar disc!" My father-in-law and brother-in-law, both orthopedic surgeons, explained that the large extruded piece of disc was compressing and displacing the major nerves to my legs, which accounted for the excruciating symptoms.

Despite the extreme discomfort, I continued to work. I actually operated for 3 weeks walking like a 100-year-old man, 1 inch at a time. I sought opinions from three distinguished back surgeons, who all agreed that a back operation was practically unavoidable. Fortunately, my sister and brother (a nurse and a physician) and my brother-in-law encouraged me to avoid surgery and to endure the pain for as long as possible.

I suffered while working during the day and said my prayers every night. I went to physical therapy, where a medieval traction machine stretched my head and legs in opposite directions. I was nearly incapacitated. Then, for no apparent reason, I awoke one morning, got out of bed, and could place my full weight on my feet with no noticeable pain in either leg. The contrast was dramatic. I could barely walk the evening before, but the very next morning, I felt normal. I wanted to break into a triumphant sprint around the house! I was ecstatic; the unrelenting pain miraculously disappeared.

Within 1 week, I was back to hitting golf balls and vigorously exercising. Neither my medical colleagues nor I could understand how this incredible change of events had suddenly occurred, within a matter of hours. While we may never figure out an explanation, I am convinced that things that defy medical knowledge happen often. A miracle?

Let me provide another personal example. One May evening, I was biking along the Little Miami Trail in Ohio, a scenic trail that runs along a river, over meadows, and through woodlands beneath spectacular canopies of trees. As I pedaled toward a rare intersection, I saw a car approaching from the east. I was a bit annoyed because I would need to slow down, and I was already behind my 60-minute goal. The driver also slowed to a near stop, which I misinterpreted

Osher RH. *The Real ABCs: A Surgeon's Analysis and a Father's Legacy, Second Edition* (pp 125-127).

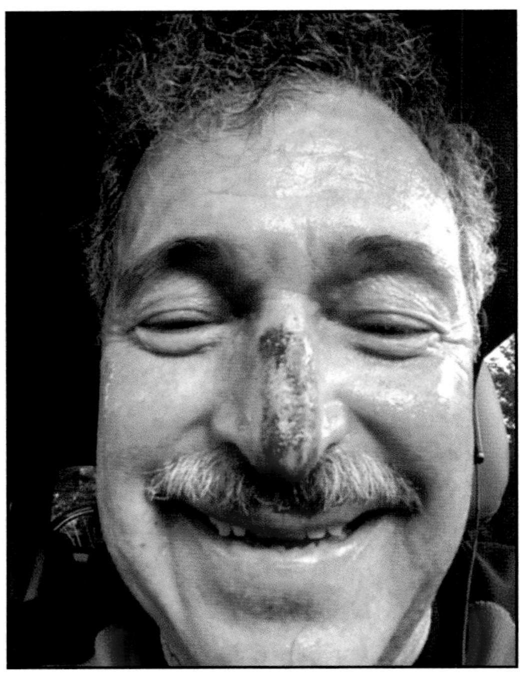

Figure 28-1. Getting hit by a car driven by a lady with cataracts!

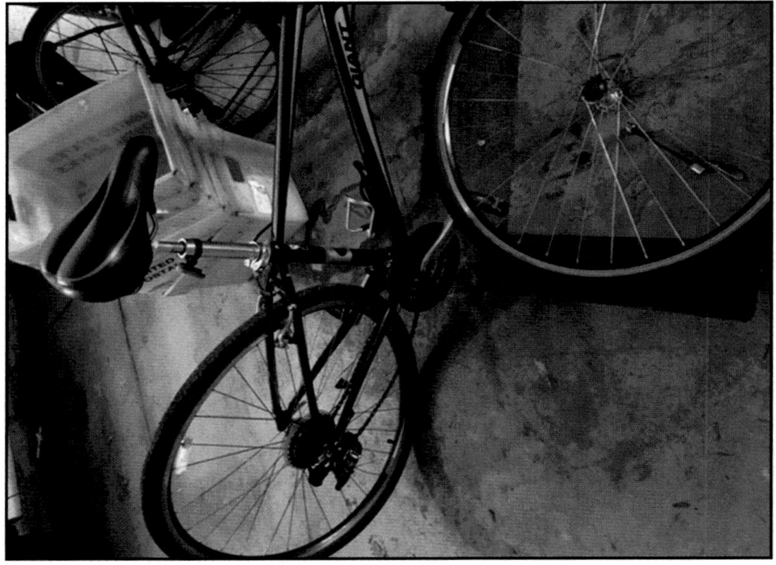

Figure 28-2. Bike pronounced dead at the scene.

as a thoughtful gesture. So, I entered the intersection only to hear the engine gunned as the car lurched forward, sending me airborne, and demolishing my bike. I landed on the concrete but was able to walk away without any major injury other than a jammed right thumb and a bloodied face (Figure 28-1). When the police arrived and saw the bike, they said that it was a miracle that I was even conscious (Figure 28-2). It turns out that the driver was an 80-year-old woman with bilateral cataracts. Heading directly into the setting sun, the glare was responsible for her not seeing me. Her insurance company replaced my bike and shattered sunglasses, allowing me to return to the trail a few days later. Perhaps I was just lucky because I could have easily been crippled, but that is another bullet I have dodged, leading me to believe that miracles never cease!

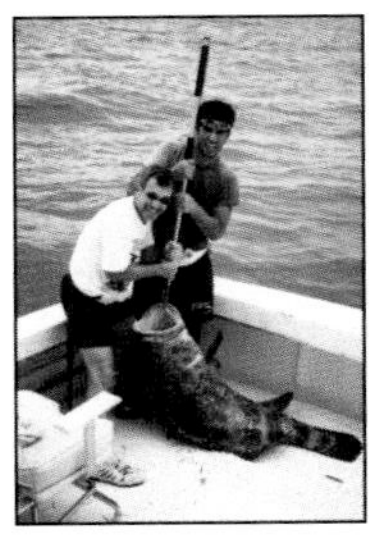

CHAPTER 29

Philanthropy

Achievement is not just limited to personal accomplishments. The act of "giving back" should also be viewed as an achievement, even though it may be very private and personal. Those who achieve their career goals are often rewarded by substantial wealth, which can be used to support a variety of worthwhile causes. However, I have never believed that it is the total number of dollars given that measures philanthropy. There are many good souls who accomplish a great deal with just their hearts and their time.

When I returned to Cincinnati, Ohio to begin my surgical practice, I decided to select several groups to which I would try to donate my time, as well as some dollars. I figured that most of the large charities had plenty of wealthy donors, and my smaller contribution would be much less significant. I had an obvious soft spot for children, so I decided to financially sponsor multiple youth basketball and baseball teams. Some of the teams only required uniforms, and this was quite inexpensive. Other teams composed of older kids who were traveling to distant tournaments were much more costly. I was surprised to learn that when one adds up the cost of uniforms, basketballs, food, transportation, hotels, etc, the bills for a team would often exceed $10,000. The cost, however, was small compared to the pleasure that I derived from not only sponsoring the teams, but eventually serving as an avid and passionate coach.

Because I had been exposed to the Big Brothers Organization during college, I decided to reach out to the Cincinnati group. There were actually several divisions in Cincinnati, including Big Sisters, so I made a commitment to invite several hundred children and their mentors for an annual riverboat ride on the Ohio River. Every summer for 2 decades, I looked forward to renting a gigantic riverboat and sitting back to enjoy several hours of total chaos (Figure 29-1)! At the conclusion of the cruise, my own children would help pass out gifts, which I would purchase in bulk from a dear friend in the toy business, Corky Steiner. My basement was always loaded with boxes filled with footballs, Frisbees, trucks, teddy bears, and, of course, baseball cards. One summer, we passed out 500 tennis balls which, by the end of the afternoon, had transformed the murky Ohio River into the Yellow River!

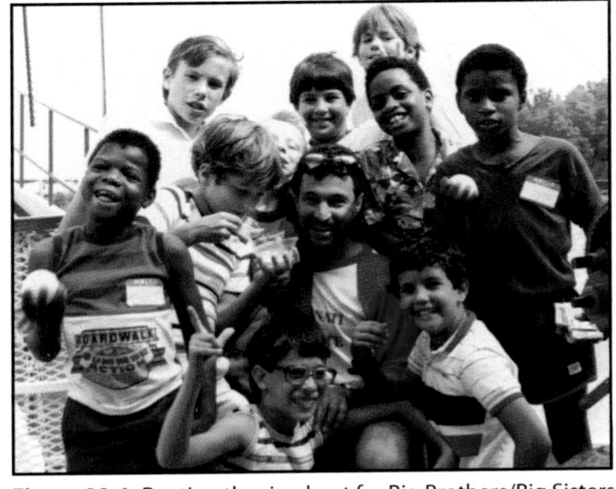

Figure 29-1. Renting the riverboat for Big Brothers/Big Sisters.

Osher RH. *The Real ABCs: A Surgeon's Analysis and a Father's Legacy, Second Edition* (pp 129-133).

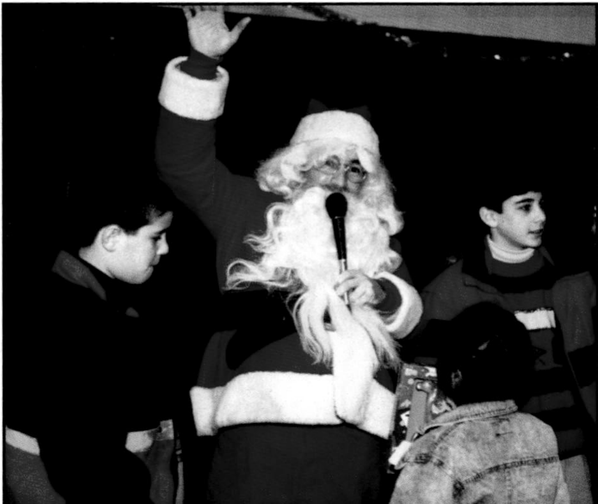

Figure 29-2. Santa with my elves, Jeff and Jamey, at the annual Beech Acres Christmas party.

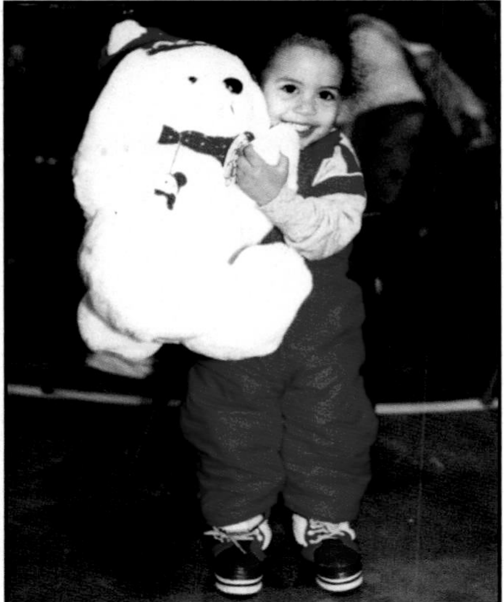

Figure 29-3. This is what it's all about!

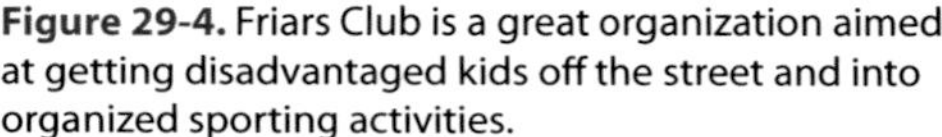

Figure 29-4. Friars Club is a great organization aimed at getting disadvantaged kids off the street and into organized sporting activities.

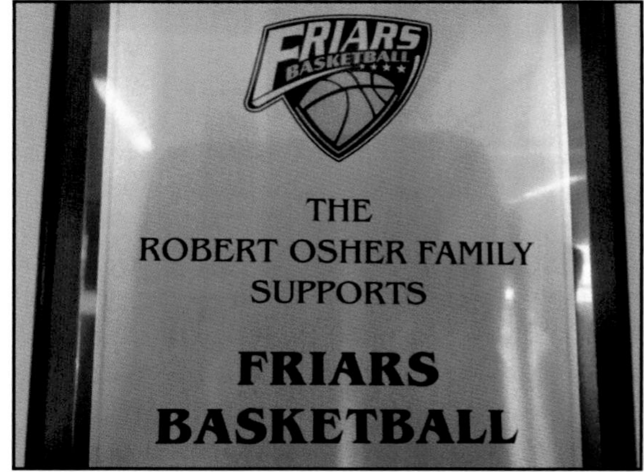

I was fortunate to learn about another magnificent organization, Beech Acres. Their mission was to care for homeless, abused, and disadvantaged children. When I found out that they needed a sponsor for their annual Christmas party, I jumped at the opportunity. In addition to sponsoring the party, I would dress up as Santa and ask my own kids to serve as elves passing out presents (Figure 29-2). With the exception of tasting Santa's beard for weeks, I found these parties, which I sponsored for years, to be very satisfying. Sometimes, the twinkle in a child's eye would bring a tear to mine (Figure 29-3).

There are many ways to express philanthropy, and my own personal preference is to avoid media attention. I have reluctantly accepted small plaques, but one of my only requests to these organizations was that there would be no publicity. It always seemed to me that any news coverage might somehow contaminate the intent. In addition to Beech Acres and the Big Brothers/Big Sisters groups, I found other worthwhile organizations dedicated to serving children. The Friars Club has a long history devoted to mentoring and providing sports programs to inner-city children. Their dedicated director, Annie Timmons, often calls when the club is encountering financial difficulties, and I do whatever I can to help. This year, I was able to contribute by covering the costs to resurface their basketball courts (Figure 29-4).

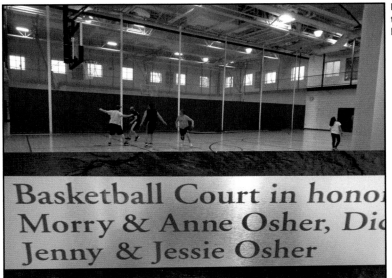

Figure 29-5. Dedication of the Jewish Community Center basketball court.

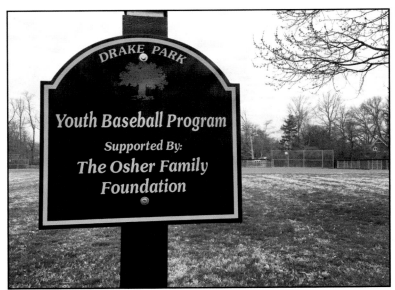

Figure 29-6. Renovation of youth baseball fields.

The American Society of Cataract and Refractive Surgery has a pediatric foundation dedicated to building eye care facilities for the indigent in Africa. I was eager to raise money for this organization by donating an unlimited number of my children's books and participating in a series of book signings. Every penny from the sales was donated, and the amount of money raised was quite significant.

As my savings account grew, I was able to do a little more. For example, when the Jewish Community Center needed a new gym for youth leagues, I joined my best friend, Bob Brant, in donating a regulation basketball court (Figure 29-5). After all, it was the experience from team sports that had shaped my life far more than anything I had ever learned in the classroom.

A local community was attempting to upgrade their youth baseball fields, and I was privileged to cover the expense, knowing that it is better to be playing ball than video games (Figure 29-6).

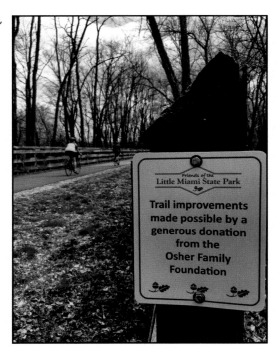

Figure 29-7. Our bike trail, the longest in the United States, needed help.

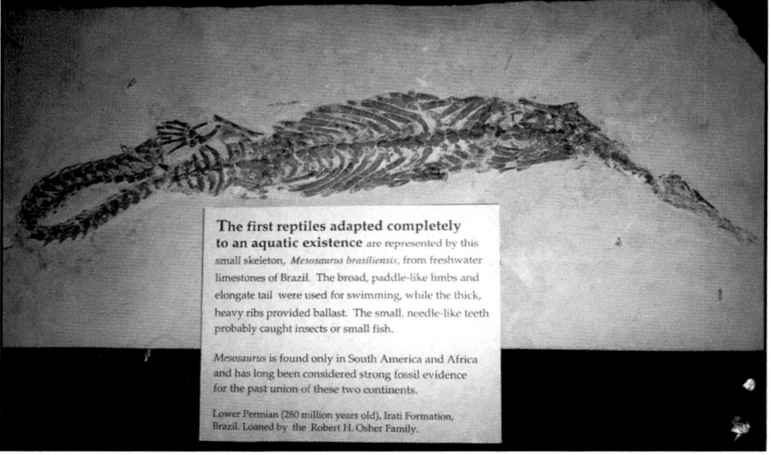

Figure 29-8. A perfectly preserved Mesosaurus, which I brought back from an excavation in Brazil and offered to the Cincinnati Museum Center.

Our local bike trail was in desperate need of structural and safety improvements, and I was fortunate to donate the funds necessary to facilitate these changes (Figure 29-7).

The renowned Cincinnati Museum Center was introducing a dinosaur exhibit and I was given the opportunity to donate a near perfectly preserved Mesosaurus, a mere 280 million years old (Figure 29-8). I've also been committed to underwriting meeting expenses for our young physicians who are training to become ophthalmologists. When it comes to the usual worthwhile charities that serve the underprivileged, those with medical needs, or necessary disaster relief, we established a small foundation that makes yearly donations. I always ask my children to select their favorite charities so that they are able to participate.

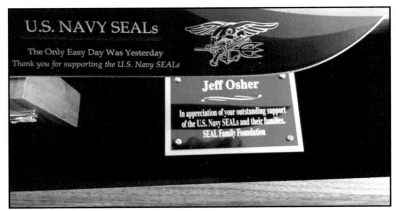

Figure 29-9. So proud of my eldest son, Jeff.

While in San Francisco, California earlier this year, I noted that my eldest son was wearing a t-shirt that supported the Navy Seals Foundation. Across the back was written, "Supporting the families of those who protect our families." I am proud that he has taken on the voluntary position to chair this worthwhile cause (Figure 29-9). In my will, I have put a portion of my life savings into a fund for my children to be able to continue "giving back" to meaningful causes.

Lastly, I want to recognize my late father, who was responsible for a longstanding philosophy that he shared when I joined him in practice. He always emphasized that, because it was a privilege to practice medicine, a physician "should not try to get rich off the ills of others." I have always felt privileged to help others, and it is a shame that my father's philosophy has almost become extinct. When a patient could not afford my services, I was always willing to provide free care. Whenever one of my senior citizens could not afford a deductible or a balance, I never hesitated to overlook it rather than place a financial strain or burden upon an elderly person. Even after I learned that my policy was illegal under the Medicare system, I continued to exercise my right to take care of needy patients and either waive balances or reduce charges whenever the patient expressed financial concerns. I try my best to give each patient excellent care, just as my father gave me excellent advice.

If we place philanthropy on our radar screen early in life, we can achieve good things for others while contributing to our sense of Contentment.

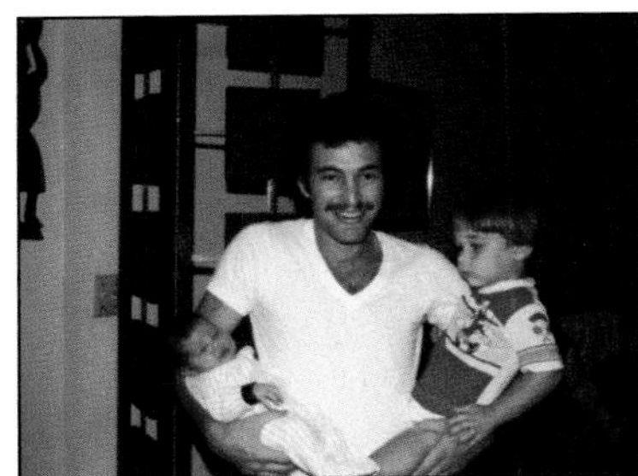

CHAPTER 30

Diversification

A Career and Recreational Strategy

For many years, I have heard the phrase, "Variety is the spice of life."* It may be more accurately stated that "diversity is the spice of life!" Perhaps I was influenced by my father, who once told me that he could never retire because he had neither interests nor hobbies outside of medicine. Few of us fully explore the broad spectrum of enjoyable diversions existing in both the workplace and in the recreational pursuits that are capable of enhancing the quality of our lives.

One of the reasons I chose ophthalmology was that this specialty included a medical practice with diverse surgical procedures. It dealt with many different diagnoses and many different treatments applicable to youngsters, as well as to senior citizens, most of whom could be helped. In other words, the diversity of the field was very attractive and allowed me to focus on what I enjoyed most—cataract surgery (Figure 30-1).

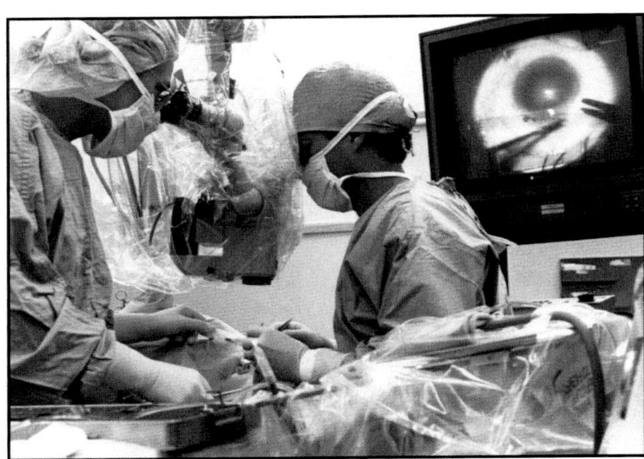

Figure 30-1. I still enjoy operating just as much as I did when I started 40 years ago when this photo was taken.

Once I began my practice, I continued to diversify my professional interests. In addition to my first priority of patient care, I allocated time for teaching. This encompassed lecturing, publishing, and producing educational videos. It was very satisfying to "give back," and it is easy to understand why so many choose an academic career that offers a lifetime of teaching. My unrelenting efforts were eventually rewarded with a professorship in the Department of Ophthalmology at the University of Cincinnati in Ohio (Figure 30-2) and recognition both within and outside of the United States (Figure 30-3).

The theme of diversification led me to found the *Audiovisual Journal of Cataract and Implant Surgery* (Figure 30-4). While incredibly time consuming and labor intensive, I have enjoyed serving as the Editor for viewers in more than 150 countries for three-and-a-half decades. My interest in video education continued to expand into the international surgery video competitions,

* William Cowper, *The Task*, 1785

Osher RH. *The Real ABCs: A Surgeon's Analysis and a Father's Legacy, Second Edition* (pp 135-144).

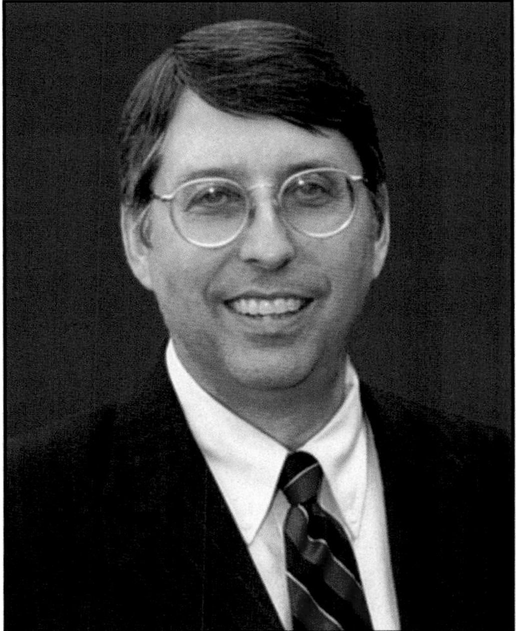

Figure 30-2. James Augsburger, MD, former Chairman of the Department of Ophthalmology, turned the residency into a first-class program.

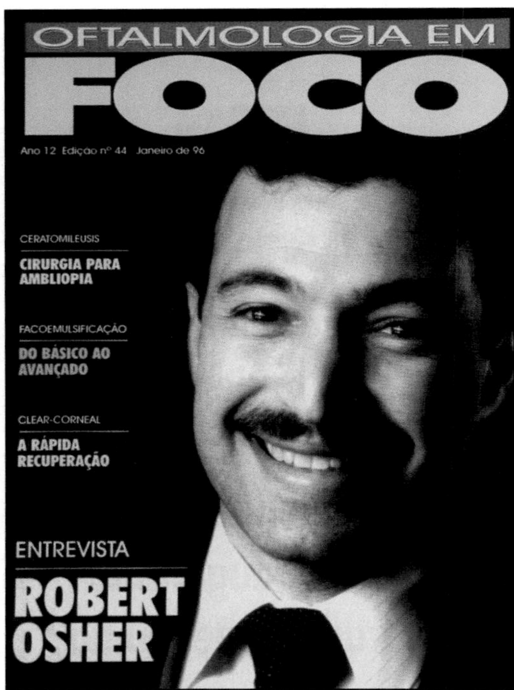

Figure 30-3. Cover of *FOCO*, a surgical magazine in Brazil.

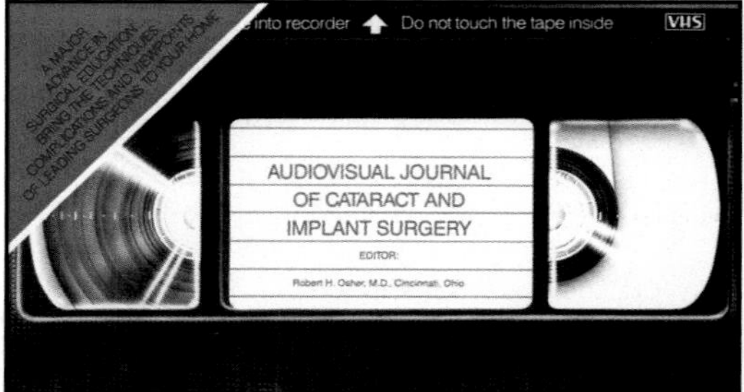

Figure 30-4. The first image *Journal* in medicine published on half-inch tape in 1985.

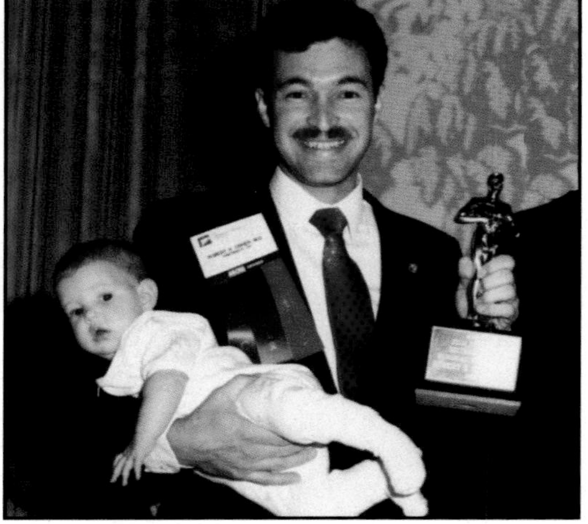

Figure 30-5. A proud winner holding two trophies!

another wonderful diversification (Figure 30-5). While it has been satisfying to be recognized with awards and prizes, the additional knowledge that I have gained by watching the surgical videos of competitors has been invaluable.

Perhaps because of these various academic endeavors, I was invited to serve on the editorial boards of multiple magazines and journals. Having a chance to review manuscripts describing new techniques kept me on the "cutting edge," usually a benefit for my patients. In addition, a number of ophthalmic companies offered consulting opportunities, which allowed me to

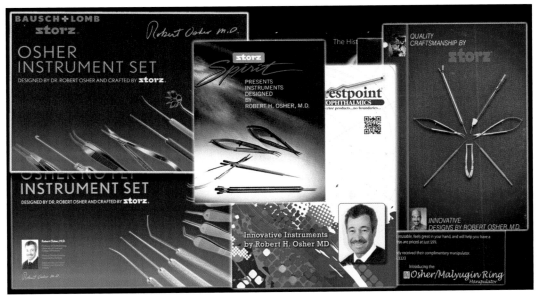

Figure 30-6. Working with industry leaders on the design and development of new surgical instruments.

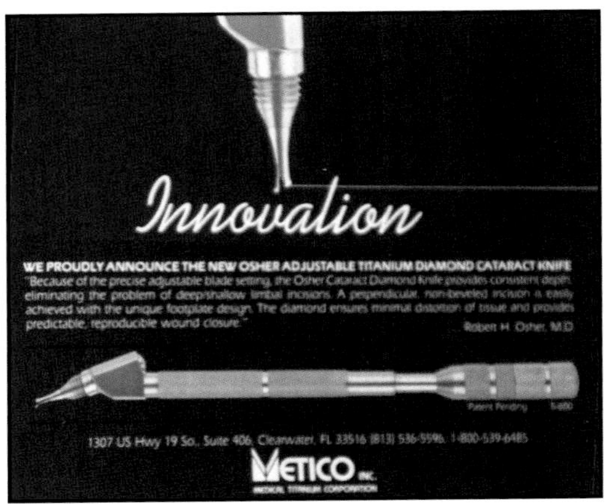

Figure 30-7. This diamond knife in the early 1980s was the first of its kind for constructing the incision.

investigate new technologies in the field of cataract surgery. I have dedicated a great deal of time to designing new instruments (Figure 30-6), lenses, and devices (Figures 30-7 and 30-8) for eye surgery, and it has been thrilling to help develop products that have contributed to a better and safer operation.

Several of the larger companies requested my assistance with their education projects, so I started a video production company that would cater to the industry. This was distinctly different than the mission of the *Video Journal of Cataract and Refractive Surgery* because it focused on new products. I was given full editorial reign and managed to film prestigious surgeons in a number of humorous situations since the most effective instruction should also be entertaining. Moreover, I had a great deal of fun creating and producing *International Advances in Phacoemulsification* and the *Video Textbook of Viscosurgery*, two perennial series featuring leading surgeons from around the world (Figure 30-9).

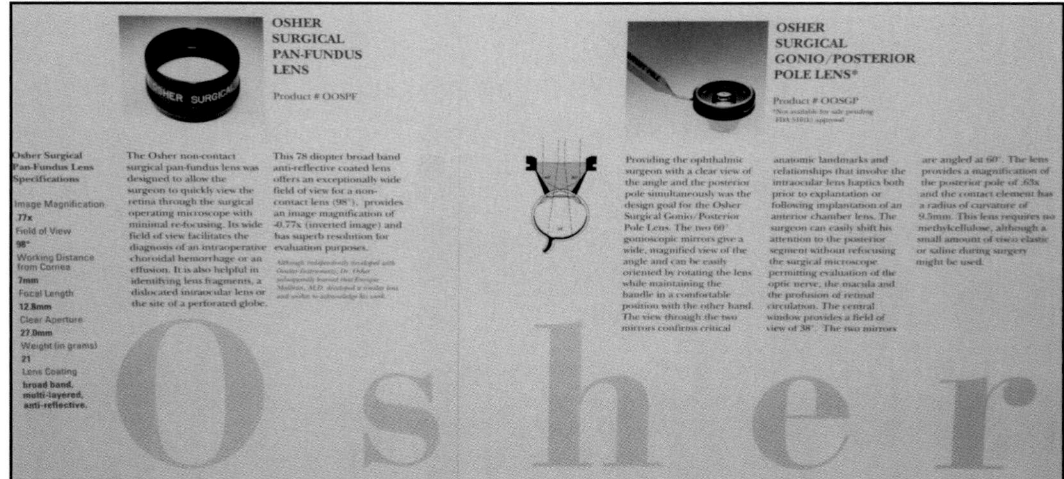

Figure 30-8. A company brochure featuring a series of surgical lenses designed to visualize places difficult to see during cataract surgery.

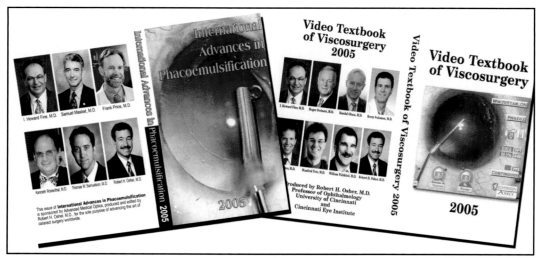

Figure 30-9. Unlike the *Video Journal*, *International Advances in Phacoemulsification* and the *Video Textbook of Viscosurgery* feature specific surgical products.

My career continued to diversify when attorneys began to call, requesting expert opinions in litigation related to cataract surgery. Since I had built my reputation on teaching the management of challenging and complicated cases, I was probably viewed as potential ammunition in these malpractice cases. What the attorneys did not expect was that I would only defend an ophthalmologist if he was innocent. I simply refused to protect an ophthalmologist who had engaged in wrongdoing, just as I refused to testify in favor of a patient suing an ophthalmologist who had acted competently in the patient's best interest. I must admit that I found the legal gymnastics, especially the depositions, quite challenging. I suspect that the lawyers would also feel challenged if they tried to perform microscopic cataract surgery!

Just like there are so many interests that one can pursue within a professional career, there are even more possibilities that fall under the category of recreational hobbies. All of my life, I have loved competitive sports and fitness. From ages 18 to 60, I would enthusiastically run a

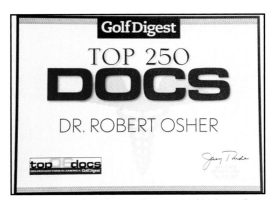

Figure 30-10. When this certificate arrived in the mail from *Golf Digest*, I thought it was a prank from my golf buddies!

NAME OSHER ROBERT GHIN. a USGA service
CLUB THE RIDGE CLUB
CLUB # 11-011 GHIN # 2126-832
EFFECTIVE DATE 10/15/08
SCORES POSTED 33 USGA HCP INDEX 5.8
C.H.: 7

SCORE HISTORY — MOST RECENT FIRST

1	78 *	77C*	79C*	79 *	78C*
6	74C*	81C	80A	78 *	78C*
11	80A	80	79A*	80C	80C*
16	84A	89A	87A	88A	89A

Figure 30-11. Universal rule: Practice makes (almost) perfect.

few miles or play a competitive game of tennis. It wasn't until I reached my 50s that my abused knees required surgical intervention, at which point I began kayaking, biking, swimming, and weightlifting. One of my best decisions was to hire a personal trainer, who pushed me to the limit during our 90-minute sessions. Under his direction, I was able to put up a valiant fight, resisting the aging process.

At age 53, I began teaching myself the game of golf, and by the end of my first year, I had read 25 books and reached my goal of shooting in the 80s. The kidney ordeal delayed my next goal of becoming a single-handicap golfer, which I later achieved in my second year. *Golf Digest* ranked me among the top physician golfers in America (Figure 30-10) and my handicap dropped to a 5 on our short 6000-yard course (Figure 30-11). Since I hit the ball like a 60-year-old woman, I like to joke with my friends when I tell them that I do my Christmas shopping from the Ladies PGA catalogue!

I must confess to a history of tennis fanaticism. After my second year of medical school, I was awarded a fellowship grant, which I used to study at the renowned Bascom Palmer Eye Institute in Miami, Florida. Every afternoon, I would hurry to the University of Miami track for a good work out. The track was located next to the tennis courts where the nationally ranked women's tennis team was practicing. I had a crush on one of the girls and decided to learn the game. She and several teammates would hit with me for hours, and I was hooked. Poor Dr. Guy O'Grady, who generously let me stay in his home, would hear balls thumping against his garage door all night long! Within several months, I could compete evenly with the girls, and it was not long before I was accepted into an elite circle of players who had competed for their college teams. I met such great people through tennis, such as world famous retinal surgeon, Dr. Harry Flynn in Miami. "Moonlighting" for room and board as a tennis teacher during my Fellowship in Philadelphia, Pennsylvania, I gave weekly lessons to Dr. Jerry Shields, an internationally renowned ophthalmic oncologist. Can you imagine the thrill of hitting respectable ground strokes with Wimbledon champion Ken Rosewall (Figure 30-12)? For the next 10 years, I worked out weekly with All-American Karen Kippley, and shortly before a career-ending wrist injury, won a Cincinnati Pro-Am tournament with Xavier and University of Cincinnati tennis coach, Eric Toth (Figure 30-13). I even had the pleasure of playing on center court at UCLA with three-time all-American Joni Urban, and was invited to introduce her when she was inducted into the Hall of Fame.

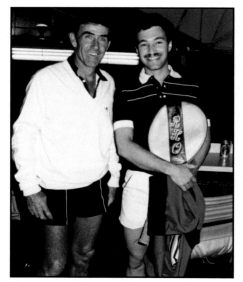

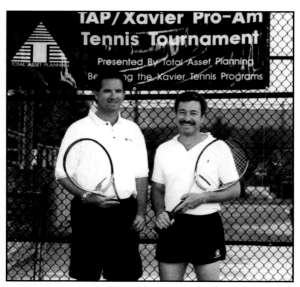

Figure 30-12. Hitting with Ken Rosewall was a real thrill.

Figure 30-13. Xavier University and University of Cincinnati tennis coach and collegiate star, Eric Toth.

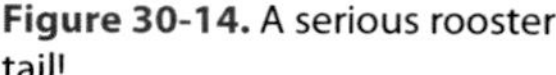

Figure 30-14. A serious rooster tail!

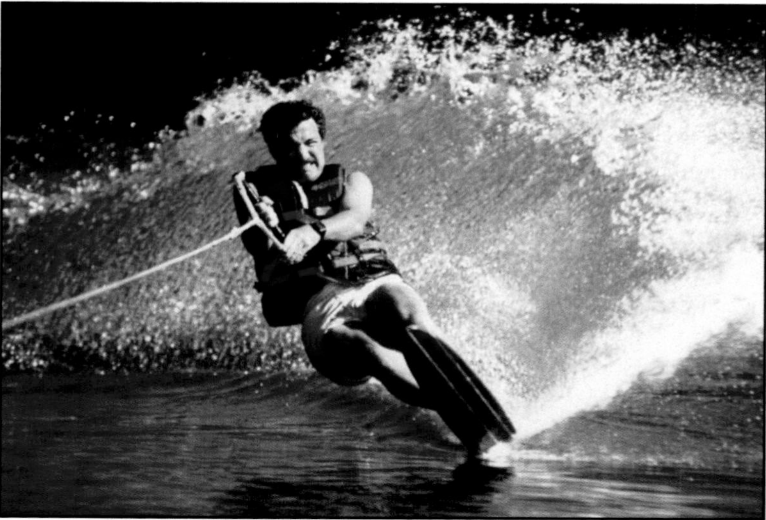

I was also hooked on slalom and trick skiing, which I taught myself by reading a library book (Figure 30-14). I would ski on canoe paddles, broomsticks, and just about anything that would float. Being on the water was always magical for me. Debbie and I celebrate my birthday every year by flying to Winnipeg and taking a tiny plane 600 miles north to a remote lake in the Canadian wilderness. We just love being in "God's country," inhabited only by bears, moose, eagles, loons, wolves, and monster Northern Pike (Figure 30-15). If we don't catch fish, we don't eat!

Incidentally, I even proposed to Debbie when we were fishing. While I was catching nothing, she had just landed yet another big fish, at which point she announced that it was time for her morning tea. As she opened her thermos, I changed her lure to a big frog and slipped the diamond ring through the frog's nose. Moments later, I predicted, "Honey, this lure is guaranteed

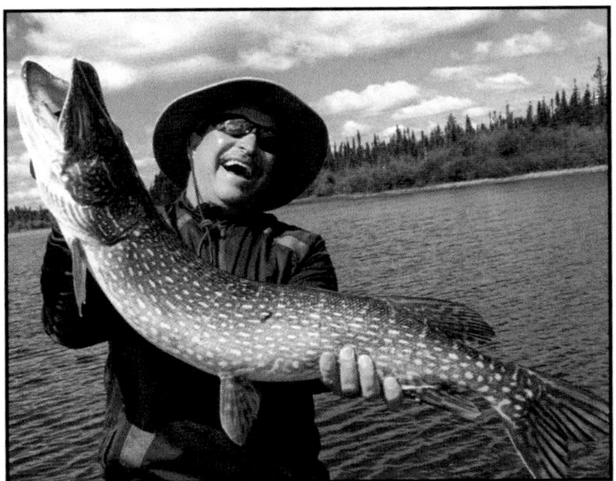

Figure 30-15. Now that is a big Pike!

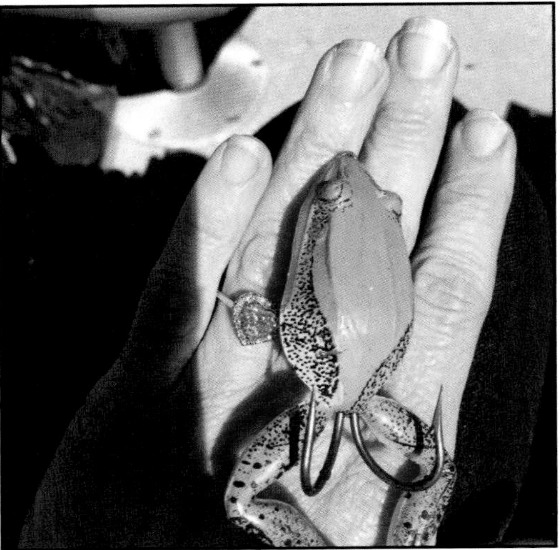

Figure 30-16. One expensive lure!

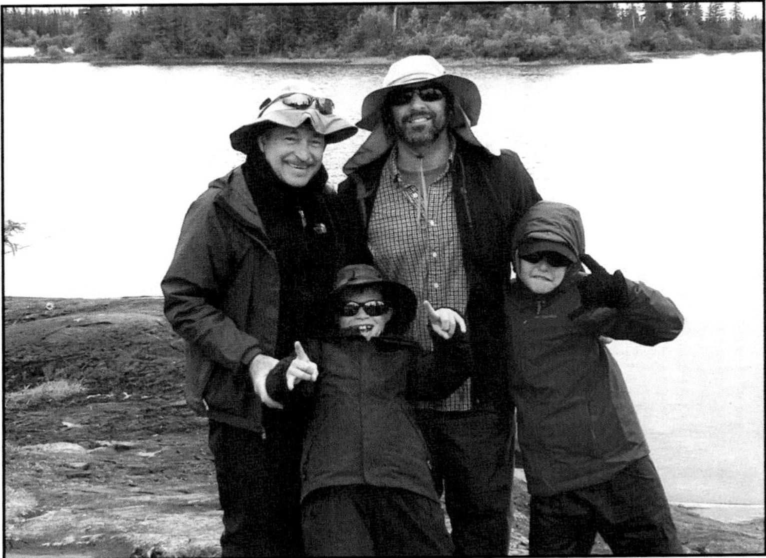

Figure 30-17. Three generations of fishermen.

to bring you a trophy!" I cast the frog out about 50 yards and handed her the rod. As Debbie began retrieving the line, it suddenly occurred to me that a monster Pike with razor-sharp teeth could cut the line and swallow the ring, turning my romantic proposal into a total catastrophe, or maybe the ring would snag the weeds and snap the line. I took a deep breath and decided it was up to fate. Her retrieval must have inspired the inventor of slow-motion movies, and after an eternity, the frog made it safely back into our small boat. As she gazed at the shiny reflection in the frog's mouth, she suddenly realized that the mysterious object was a ring. She jumped up, nearly tipping the boat, and blurted, "Yes, I do!" before I could even pop the question. We embraced, kissed, and the frog did not turn into a handsome prince. However, the ring was safe, the princess was hooked, and I reminded her that I kept my promise about the trophy (Figure 30-16)! We recently took three generations of Oshers back to our favorite fishing venue, and it was so satisfying to see that my grandsons will continue this tradition (Figure 30-17).

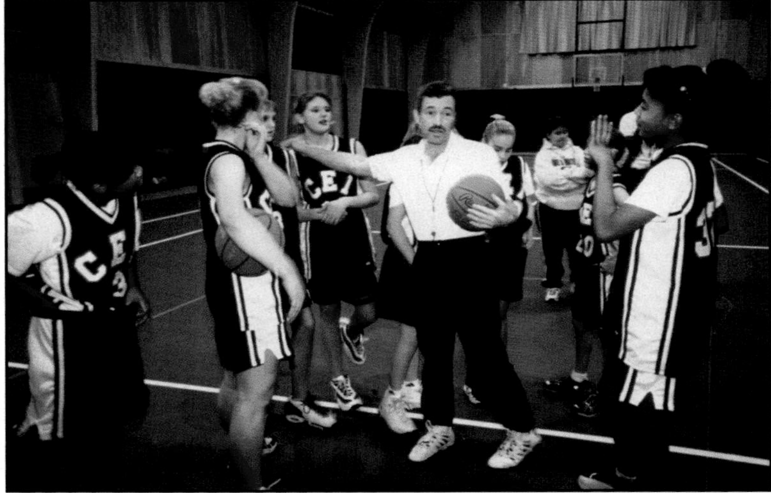

Figure 30-18. While I love teaching elite athletes, I have learned that only the girls listen!

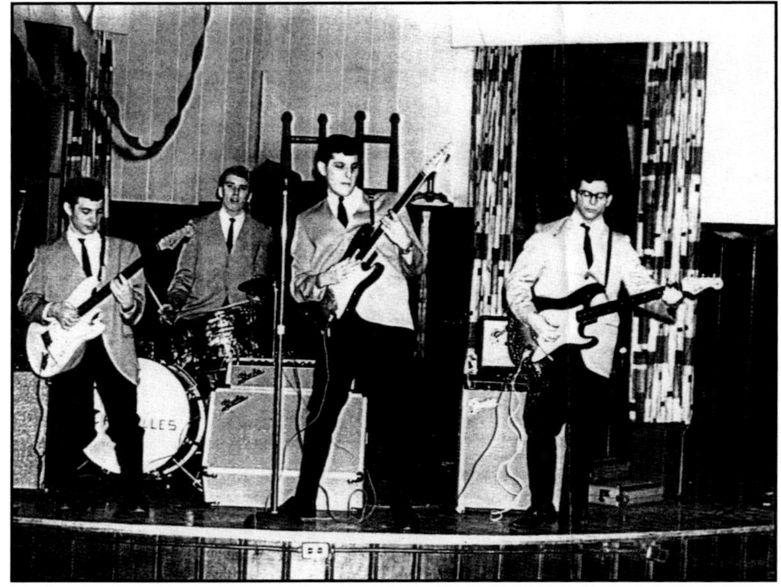

Figure 30-19. In case you are wondering, that is not Eric Clapton on the left.

Coaching has also been fantastic hobby, and more than 70 baseball and basketball teams have endured my tough but dedicated style (Figure 30-18). If my hands ever start to shake in the operating room, a career in coaching would certainly be an attractive alternative!

There are so many other exhilarating hobbies besides sports that make life incredibly enjoyable. Music is a wonderful pastime, which in my case began in a rock band in high school (Figure 30-19). Before my children were born, I could not wait to play bass on weekend nights at Crockett's, a river boat where one of my high school friends, Ernie Waits, had assembled a talented group of musicians to provide the night club entertainment (Figure 30-20). However, arriving home at 3:00 am with a surgery schedule the next morning did not last long! Instead, I bought a keyboard and composed funny songs for the kids, which we would sing together at bedtime (Figure 30-21). I still enjoy listening to music every evening when I am exercising or preparing my surgical charts for the next day.

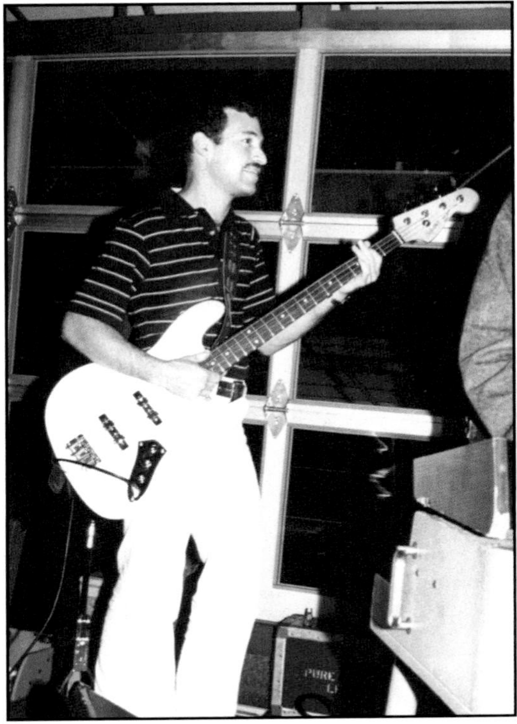

Figure 30-20. I had to stop playing bass guitar all night long because my fingertips were numb, and I was deaf the next day in the operating room!

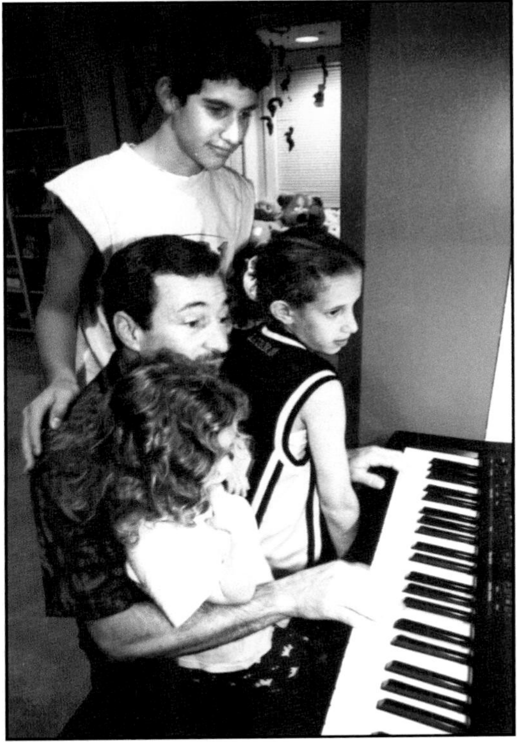

Figure 30-21. I placed a keyboard in each bedroom so we could sing together before the children fell asleep.

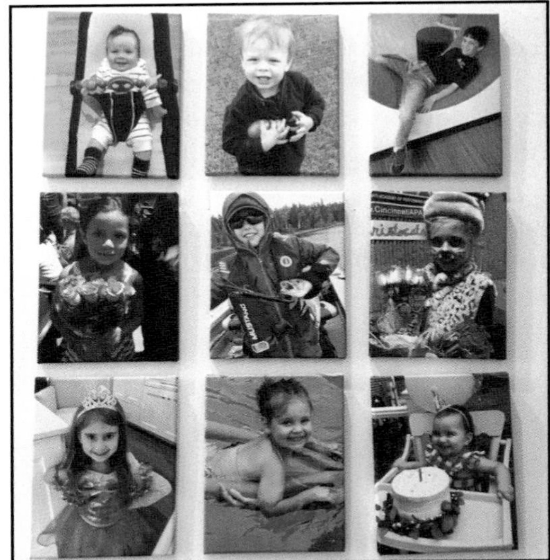

Figure 30-22. I love taking pictures of grandchildren.

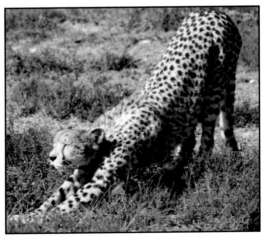

Figure 30-23. Our walls are covered with wildlife photography.

Card magic was another area that held my interest when I was in medical school. I would frequently entertain the children on the pediatric wards, making cards mysteriously disappear and temporarily lifting their spirits in a depressing place from which I wished the children could disappear. Gardening, fishing, diving, and photography (Figures 30-22 and 30-23) have each

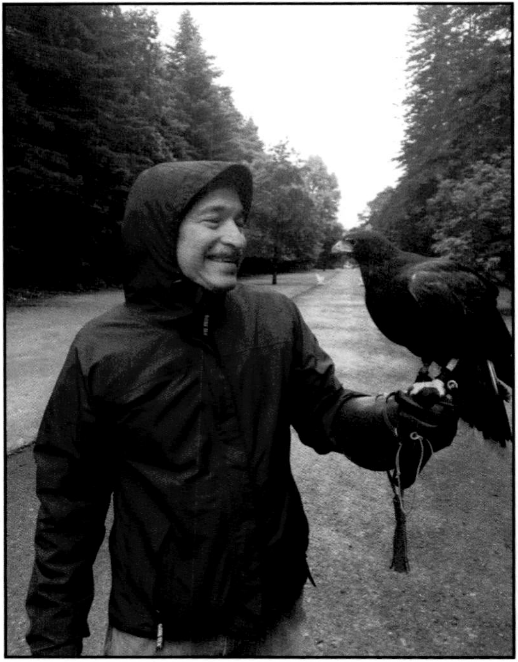

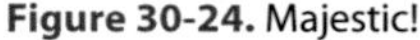
Figure 30-24. Majestic!

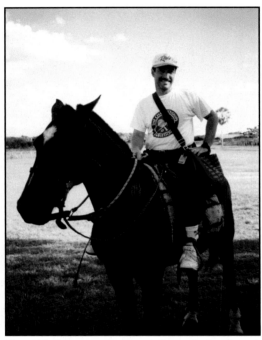

Figure 30-25. I am not Roy Rogers, but galloping through the Pantanal in Brazil is the only way to go!

enriched my life. I have even enjoyed hawking in England (Figure 30-24) and birdwatching in the Brazilian Pantanal on horseback (Figure 30-25).

The message is really quite simple. Our lives offer limited time to take advantage of a countless number of satisfying activities, both in our careers and in our recreational free time. I feel sadness every time I see a kid planted on the couch held hostage by the television or mesmerized by either a computer game or cell phone. The clock is ticking for each of us, and I never want to look back with regret and say, "I wish I had done this or that."

What is the universal antidote for boredom or depression? Stay busy! What is the best medicine for maintaining interest and enthusiasm? Stay active! Life is not a dress rehearsal. I believe that career and recreational diversification are the keys to enjoying life to its fullest.

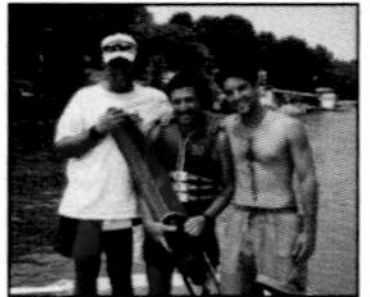

CHAPTER 31

Thoughts About Aging

I am fortunate to interact with senior citizens every day because my practice is limited to cataract surgery. As a result, I have ample opportunity to observe and ask questions about the aging process on a daily basis. Patients encourage me to "smell the roses" before it is too late. Perhaps they mean that we should not delay gratification, or maybe they mean that all senses, including the sense of smell, will decay with age. Patients also tell me that the "golden years" are not very golden, but, as many have said before me, aging certainly beats the alternatives!

Like everyone, I wrestle with the consequences of age, and I like to joke that my photographic memory no longer develops. I can walk into the operating room, receive greetings from the nurses and technicians with whom I have worked closely for years, then suddenly draw a blank on one of their names. This is really awful. While I used to be able to run like a deer with effortless endurance, I find myself breathing heavily when I ascend the stairs to my third-floor office. Although I still have my original hair, I seem to have much more face to wash! As an ophthalmologist, I still curse the fact that I cannot see much of anything up close without my $5 reading glasses, which I either misplace or lose every day (which explains the price). On the golf course, I have transitioned from the member tees to the senior tees, and lately I am considering a final move to the women's tees! Even the professional baseball and basketball players on TV look like they should still be in high school. Probably, some of them should be.

So many brilliant writers have made highly intelligent and philosophical observations about aging, but I am not looking for the Fountain of Youth, nor am I interested in trying to fool anyone with cosmetic surgery. I am, however, trying to wage a respectable battle with Father Time in order to age gracefully. While I may be frustrated when searching for my keys and finding my misplaced wallet, the big question seems to be how to remain as emotionally and physically healthy as possible. A good mental attitude in combination with a reasonable physical aptitude is a highly desirable combination when one is on the catabolic side of life's bell-shaped curve.

A renowned eye surgeon in Beverly Hills, California, Dr. Samuel Masket, likens the aging process to a conveyor belt at Federal Express. He says that we are all like boxes of different sizes and shapes, moving in the same direction, then invariably dropping off, one after another. After hearing this analogy, I stopped using Federal Express! I suspect that many of my patients who are on multiple antidepressants spend far too much time thinking about dying, while forgetting to live. I prefer an alternative approach: live every minute as if it were your last!

Osher RH. *The Real ABCs: A Surgeon's Analysis and a Father's Legacy, Second Edition* (pp 145-148).

When I see a very happy 85-year-old patient, I often try to politely ask what factors contribute to feeling so good about life. Although the answers may vary, there seems to be a few common themes, which I will try to recount. First, it is essential to stay engaged with work, hobbies, or something that keeps the mind active. We need to look forward to awakening every day to accomplish something meaningful. When I was a second-year medical student, I was inspired by an enthusiastic, retired surgeon in his late 80s who would donate his time to helping us with our cadaver dissections in the anatomy lab. When I was a resident at Bascom Palmer Eye Institute in Miami, Florida, there was another retired physician in his 90s who volunteered as an assistant librarian. He took such great pride in being able to find just about any article that we needed for a research project or a presentation. At the Natural History Museum in Cincinnati, Ohio, there is a group of senior volunteers who run the train exhibits over the holidays. I admire their unbridled excitement when they explain the history of the railroad. These individuals stand out in my memory because they share in common a genuine happiness as a result of remaining active and doing something nice for others.

I have also noticed that my most contented seniors seem to stay connected with family or friends. They have not allowed themselves to become isolated, which worries me because I am a loner. They seem to enjoy socializing, giving credence to the philosophy that life is meant to be shared. Unfortunately, it is this same group of patients who are most devastated when they lose a spouse or close acquaintance. I am reminded by the cliché, "better to have loved and lost than never to have loved at all."*

I have also observed that patients who are happy like to laugh. They seem to have maintained their sense of humor over the years. I recall one patient with chronic iritis who would give me a big smile when he pointed to his left eye and say, "You're wrong doc, it's not eye rightis.... it's eye leftis!" Another one of my octogenarians was on the operating room table, and as I always do, I asked if he was comfortable. He replied, "Thanks for asking, doc, I make a pretty good living!" Although I do not claim to understand the biochemistry of laughter, I am sure that it is very healthy for the mind and the body to continue laughing throughout a lifetime.

From my own experiences, I have noticed that awareness of nature's abundant gifts can inject joy into a routine day. A perfect example is the majestic hawk that I observed perched on the edge of a building (Figure 31-1). An hour later, as I was taking a walk, combining a boring conference call with a little exercise, I was treated to the beauty of a tiger swallowtail enjoying a sip of nectar from a flower (Figure 31-2). Although our senses may diminish with advancing years, a deep appreciation of nature can bring a smile to any face, regardless of age.

Mundane issues like competent financial planning can also bring a sense of Contentment. I have never been a very materialistic person, and I do not own a fancy car, a boat, or fancy clothes. I have always believed that the best things in life are not things! So, I have not paid a great deal of attention to investment opportunities or schemes to make money. However, I have been committed to preserving my hard-earned nest egg. When I was young, my father taught me not to worry about the return on the principal, but rather making certain that the principal was returned. I am fortunate that my eldest son became one of the most successful hedge-fund managers in the United States, and I have been rewarded by simply trusting his good judgement and not asking questions.

* Alfred Lord Tennyson, *In Memoriam*, 1850

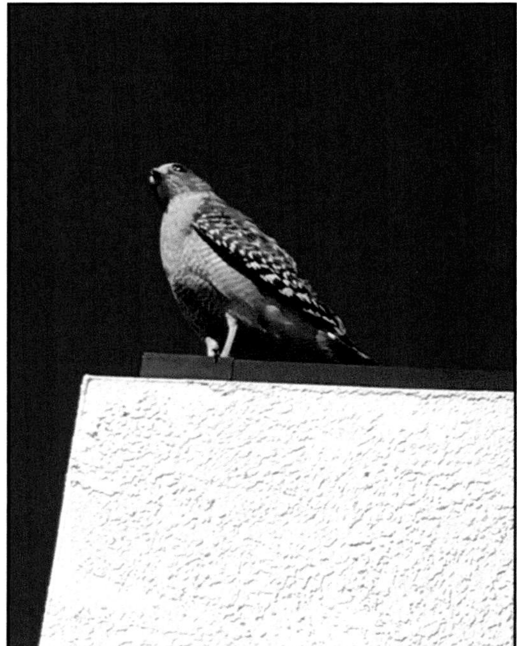
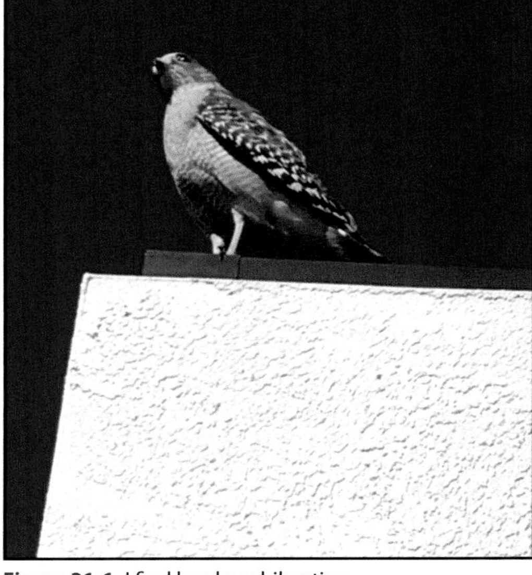

Figure 31-1. I find hawks exhilarating...

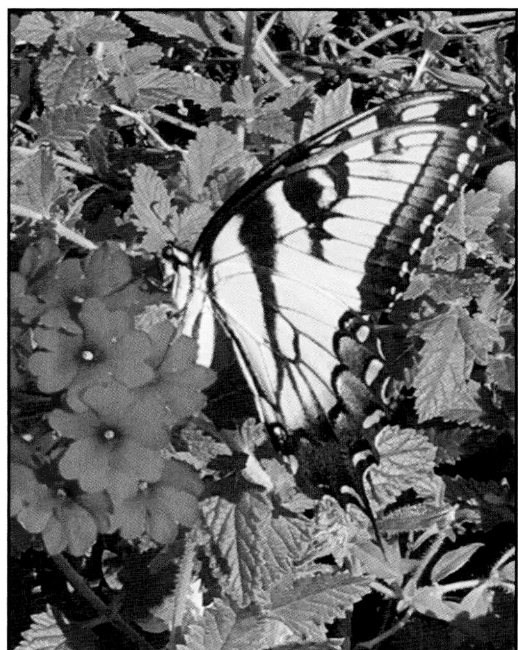

Figure 31-2. ...and butterflies are show-stoppers...

I have also observed that money can fracture business associates, close friends, and tight families. I figured that good financial planning would prevent this catastrophe from happening, so I retained the very best expert—who just happens to be my best friend since childhood, Robert Brant. From the first day of my practice, I put away the maximum legal contribution for each of my children and established lead trusts. When my children had children, I felt strongly about fully funding their 529 accounts, so my first wife, Barbara, and I could have the satisfaction of knowing that we were giving the most important gift—education—to each grandchild. While I have always been comfortable living a very simple life, the balance in my bank account gradually increased to the point where I was able to help others in addition to my children and grandchildren. One definite advantage of the aging process is that many seniors have accumulated enough wealth to be able to give back and take care of their families and others. This can be a great source of satisfaction later in life.

Finally, as we come to grips with our own mortality, I find that those who have the greatest sense of peace and Contentment have been able to find meaning in their lives. In other words, if you honestly believe that we are here for a reason, you are living your life by a different yardstick. Religious faith and a sense of purpose are powerful anecdotes to the emotional consequences of age.

In closing, I am going to reveal a personal secret that has been far better than discovering the Fountain of Youth: grandchildren (Figure 31-3)! These nine boys and girls have brought so much happiness to my life and are a monumental gift that I never anticipated. Watching these little ones grow up is truly an amazing and exhilarating experience. As a grandparent, I have the right to spoil my grandchildren, and if they misbehave, I can give them back! Seriously, I would have to rank grandchildren as the number one benefit of aging.

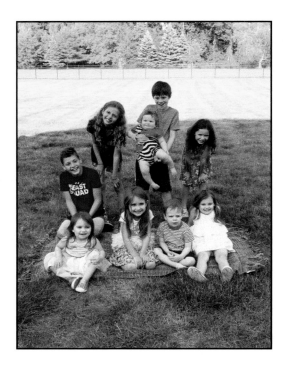

Figure 31-3. ...but nothing beats the ultimate gift—grandchildren!

Dr. Spencer Thornton, a renowned eye surgeon from Nashville, Tennessee, just celebrated his 90th birthday, and he is still as sharp as a tack. He recently told me that life is like a roll of toilet paper: the closer you get to the end, the faster it goes! So, my final advice to every reader (since we are all aging) is to make the most of every moment. Celebrate the present and look forward to tomorrow with anticipation. Someday, when you finally look back, you will have no regrets.

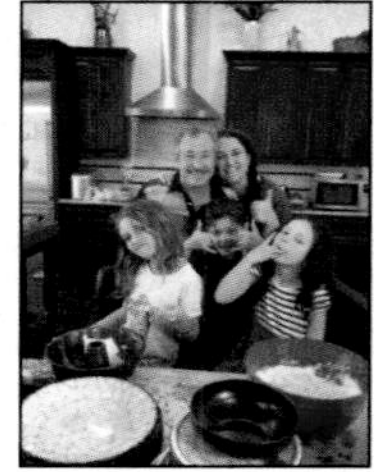

CHAPTER 32

A Second Chance

In the game of life, we are occasionally given a second chance, and sometimes not. After a whirlwind trip visiting and interviewing at a dozen medical schools, I recall on the final day, we had scheduled the very first interview at Strong Memorial Hospital at the University of Rochester. My father had also managed to secure the very last time for an interview at the Dartmouth Medical School. I honestly do not remember how we managed to get from the western side of New York State to Vermont, but I clearly recall every word of the final interview. The Dean was summarizing my candidacy by complimenting my academic performance in college, remarking about my strong letters of recommendation, and volunteering how impressed he was with my drive and discipline. When he paused, I quickly interjected with enthusiasm how much I had enjoyed the tour and how certain I was that I would become an excellent medical student at the University of Rochester. Unfortunately, I had left that property earlier that day and was interviewing at Dartmouth! Needless to say, the Dean concluded that a disoriented candidate would be better off elsewhere, and ironically, I did wind up going to medical school at the University of Rochester. Still, it would have been nice to have had a second chance to "redo" that conversation, which still haunts me to this day.

My marriage of 38 years was not going smoothly, for which I was mostly to blame. My wife, Barbara, was a beautiful, athletic, intelligent woman who married me when she was still a teenager. For decades, I was so focused on building the Cincinnati Eye Institute, developing the first subspecialty practice limited to cataract surgery by referral, and traveling the world in order to teach that I largely neglected our marriage. My usual routine consisted of a full day in surgery, rushing home to coach the kids, running for 1 hour while they were eating dinner, telling them a bedtime story or singing them to sleep, and then heading back to the office to work until the early hours of the morning. Admittedly, I was not a very good husband. My wife and I grew further and further apart, but what kept us together was a strong devotion to our children. She went to bed early, I went to bed long after midnight. She enjoyed watching TV, I viewed it as a distraction. I enjoyed traveling, but her loyalty to the kids prevented her from accompanying me. I was deeply into fitness; she was not. She loved dancing and was very good at it, while I was born with two left feet. Over time, our relationship was reduced to co-managing the children and paying the bills. I considered divorce, but I still had a very young daughter, so I hung in there. However, when two people do not invest the time to communicate nor share interests, the marriage is terminal.

Osher RH. *The Real ABCs: A Surgeon's Analysis and a Father's Legacy, Second Edition* (pp 149-155).

Everybody has the right to be happy, yet happiness is not an easy state to achieve. While I was accustomed to traveling to conferences where I would eat, exercise, and sleep alone, I often wondered if it might be more enjoyable to share life with a companion. I certainly had more fun when I used to take each of my kids to conferences with me when they were young. I would work hard teaching and then play hard with whichever child came with me. That was about the extent of my companionship.

Then came Debbie. I had known this vivacious woman for many years since she served as the Executive Director of the Connecticut Society of Eye Physicians and had invited me on several occasions to be a guest speaker for their annual meeting. I was always impressed by how she could organize a conference better than anyone I had ever met, taking care of every little detail, the speakers, the exhibitioners, and the members of her society while earning respect and appreciation from all. When she was not running this society, she was also serving as the Executive Director for the ENT; Dermatology; and surgical societies. In addition, she was a tenacious fighter in the Connecticut Senate, going nose-to-nose with anyone who tried to "dummy down" medicine. Even senators in the U.S. Congress would call her for advice and would frequently offer her a job in Washington, D.C.

Initially, I guess I was attracted by her high-energy, dynamic personality, and unwavering principles, but she also had warmth, kindness, thoughtfulness, piercing blue eyes, and a smile that made me weak in the knees. We started spending time together, and I found out that she was a cross-country runner, talented painter, wildlife photographer, guardian of Mother Nature, and fitness buff. Wherever we would go, she would be the center of attention, easily socializing with anyone and everyone, while I preferred my more reclusive behavior. She was genuinely interested in people who, in turn, were quick to ask for her help or advice, which she gave freely. It seemed that she was always reading *Newsweek* or *National Geographic* to fuel her passion for saving the planet. Her enthusiasm for nature was expansive, and her house was loaded with butterflies, crystals, moss, bird nests, flowers, feathers, three dogs, and a hatchery for live butterflies and praying mantises. Perhaps I should mention that the walls were decorated with stuffed birds from the Smithsonian, spiders and beetles, and a few prehistoric dinosaur bones. I always felt like I was in a natural history museum!

So, as my marriage was ending, I was already falling in love with a woman 15 years younger but decades wiser. She could work as hard as me, and when not working, she was dashing to the tennis court, the gym, or a fitness class, or to read to seniors in a nursing home. I admit to being attracted to that kind of energy, and when we were together, I was a bit giddy, usually laughing, and truly happy (Figure 32-1). She allowed me to become part of her life, along with two great kids that she had raised since getting a divorce from an ophthalmologist (how ironic) years before.

As I stated earlier, I have always been a reclusive person, quite content when alone, but I could not wait to be with Debbie. It was a new experience for me to travel with a companion and combine my love of teaching with my new love. I was used to flying to Argentina or New Zealand, teaching for the day, then boarding a plane back to Cincinnati. No more insanity; Debbie was teaching me the concept of Balance. After finishing my lectures, we toured the museums in New York City and London, jogged the beaches and dove together on the Great Barrier Reef in Australia (Figure 32-2), went parasailing in the Caymans (Figure 32-3), biked through the wine country in Portugal and along the aqueducts in Wales (Figure 32-4), enjoyed a safari and paragliding over Victoria Falls in Africa, climbed volcanoes in the Azores (Figure 32-5), went ziplining through the jungle in Costa Rica, boated along the channels in Copenhagen, hiked up the Alps by Lake Como in Italy, ascended Machu Picchu in Peru (Figure 32-6), kayaked down the Salt River and descended the Grand Canyon in Arizona (Figure 32-7),

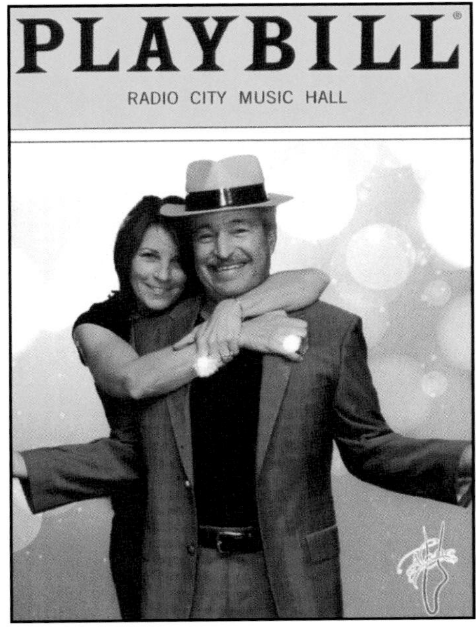

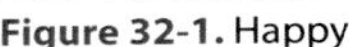
Figure 32-1. Happy!

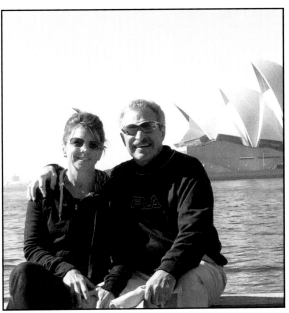

Figure 32-2. We love Australia!

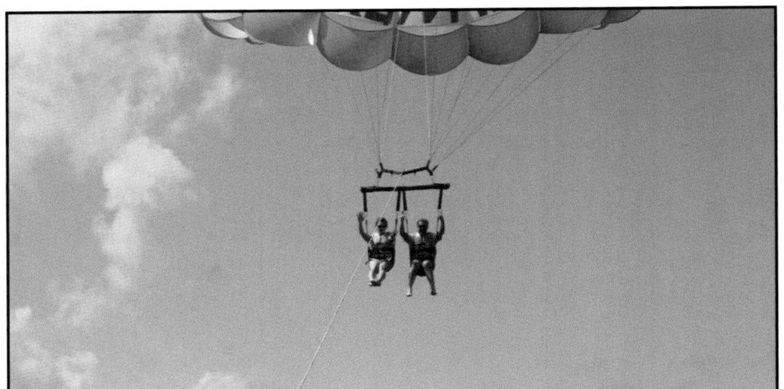

Figure 32-3. Parasailing did nothing for my fear of heights.

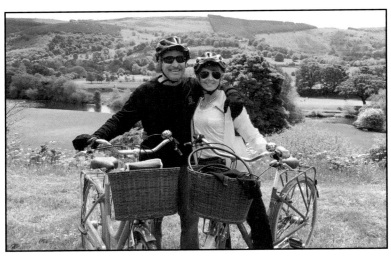

Figure 32-4. Biking together through Portugal and Wales.

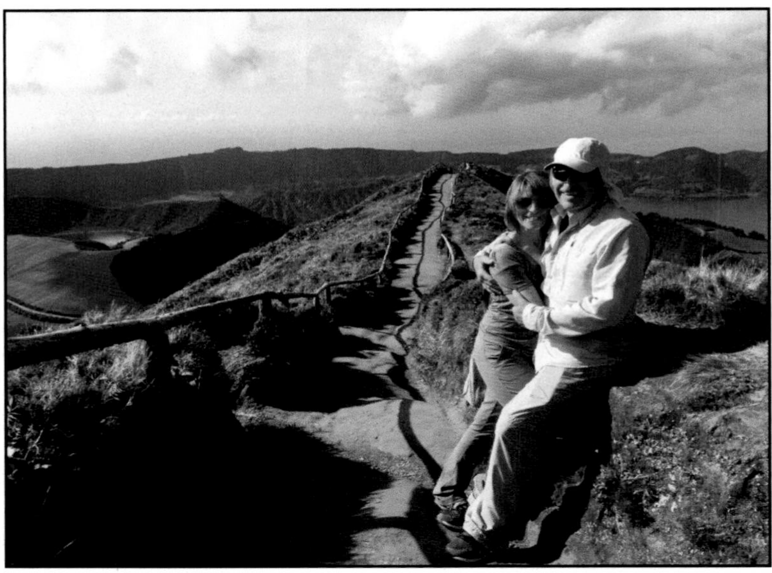

Figure 32-5. Breathtaking view from the volcano in the Azores.

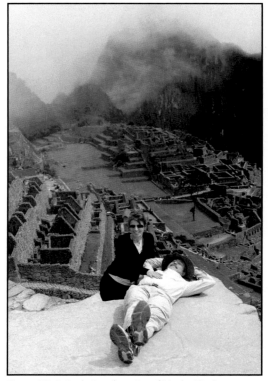

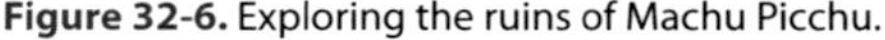

Figure 32-6. Exploring the ruins of Machu Picchu.

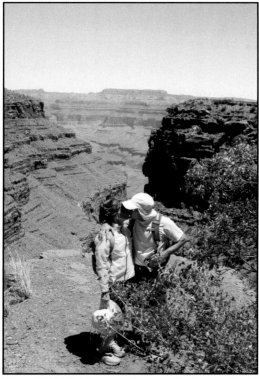

Figure 32-7. It is a long way down and back up the Grand Canyon.

visited the Taj Mahal in India (Figure 32-8), fished for Pike in Northern Canada (Figure 32-9), snowmobiled across a glacier in Iceland (Figure 32-10), chased iguanas and giant turtles in the Galapagos, explored the gorges in Slovenia (Figure 32-11) and the icebergs near Antarctica (Figure 32-12), and trekked through Patagonia and Tierra del Fuego in Chile. However, the location really

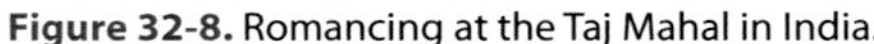 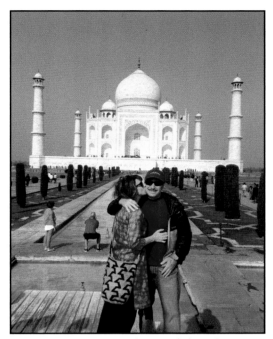
Figure 32-8. Romancing at the Taj Mahal in India.

Figure 32-10. Snowmobiling the glaciers in Iceland.

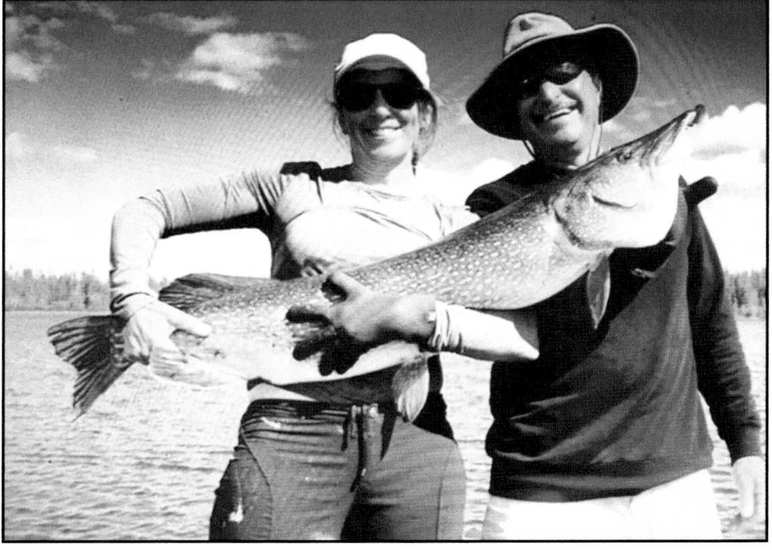

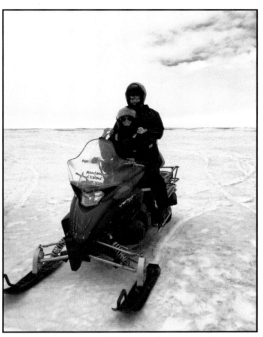
Figure 32-9. My fishing buddy.

did not matter. Big waterfall or small waterfall (Figures 32-13), we could be anywhere, and I felt joy. When we parted, I experienced an overwhelming sadness, which turned to excitement as our next rendezvous drew near. She became my closest friend, and we were perfect for each other.

With advancing age comes the wisdom to analyze the past and understand the present. Hindsight measures 20/20, and I now see how I neglected my first marriage to a very good person because I was preoccupied with my career and a burning desire to achieve. I still try to be as supportive and helpful as I can be to my first wife, and I will always care about her well-being. Moreover, I will always appreciate what a wonderful job she did raising our children. Life throws

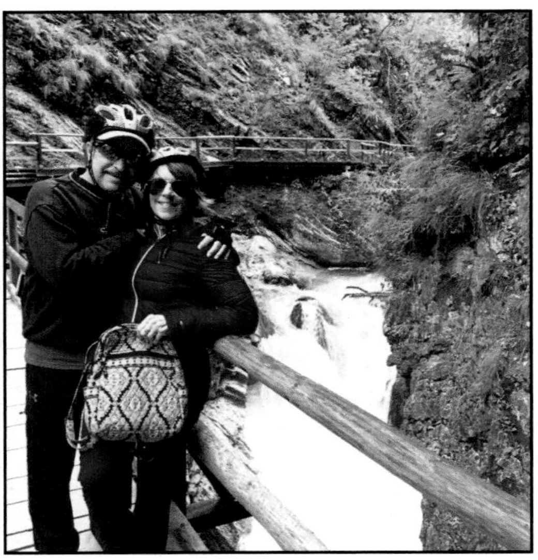

Figure 32-11. Exploring the gorges in Slovenia.

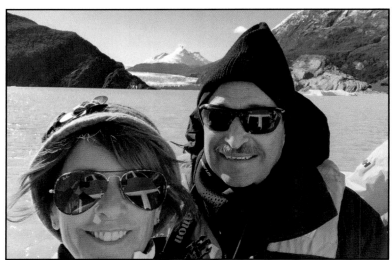

Figure 32-12. Warming up the icebergs near Antarctica.

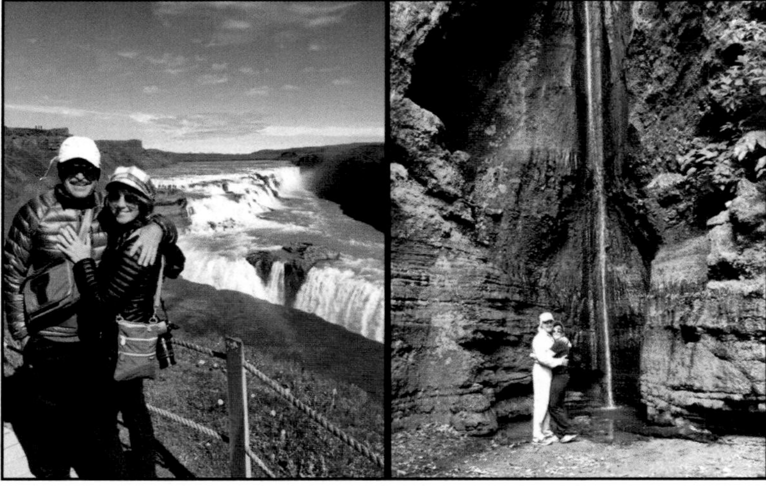

Figure 32-13. Big waterfall or small waterfall, we made a splash together.

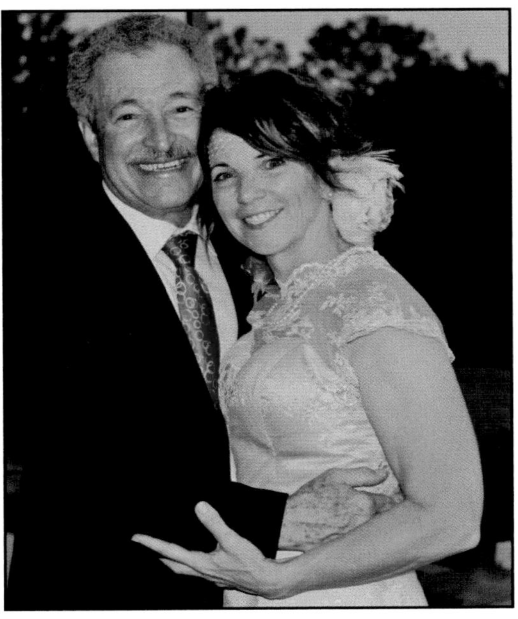

Figure 32-14. Newlyweds.

different curveballs, and although I may have struck out as a husband in my first at bat, I feel very lucky to be getting a second chance. I marvel at the way Debbie lives her life trying to save the elephants in Burma, cleaning up the beaches in Costa Rica, raising money for the injured birds in Litchfield, and saving the water supply that makes shaving my face more difficult than ever. She has also gone above and beyond, reaching out to my children and grandchildren, and she even enjoys spending time with my first wife. Debbie always inspires me, and I feel like I have become a better and more balanced person since she entered my life.

Light travels at 186,282 miles/second, yet it has taken decades to penetrate my thick skull. Finally, I am enlightened, and I see the world in shining splendor. While patient care and Achievement are still very important, my life is now devoted to another. I am deeply in love and have found Contentment. We were married on November 9, 2018, in Sarasota, Florida, surrounded by our children (Figure 32-14). Just perfect.

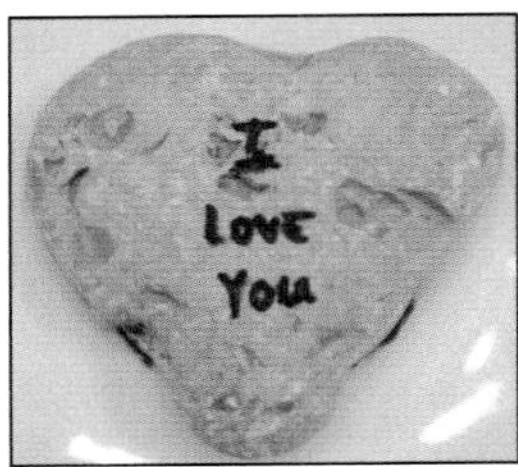

CHAPTER 33

Final Thoughts

I have always lived a very active lifestyle and have tried to cram as much as possible into each day. Yet, since my encounter with malignant kidney cancer, I have learned how to enjoy my life much more than ever before. The difference is that now I cram as much as I can into each and every day…and I appreciate every moment!

Some of the lessons that I have learned to maximize Achievement and personal happiness include the following points. First, prioritize. Figure out what is really important to achieve in your career, and then go for it. The same prioritization should apply to one's personal life.

Second, do not procrastinate or rationalize why it would be better to get started later rather than now. To put it bluntly, there may not be a later! No individual can predict the length of a lifetime, but it is a fact that every passing day is one less. Therefore, "live every day as if it were your last."*

Third, prepare for success by successful preparation. Get organized. Have a plan. Set ambitious yet realistic goals. Utilize your time efficiently and exercise the necessary discipline to stick to your program.

Fourth, relish your work. Regardless of the type of job, it should be done as well as one is capable. It is satisfying to accomplish a task, and the well-earned sense of Achievement is a great feeling!

Fifth, establish Balance in your life. Work hard and play hard. Get fit, one exercise at a time. Every so often, do something nice for somebody unrelated or for some worthwhile organization. A donation of time is every bit as satisfying as a donation of dollars. Periodically, do something adventuresome and diversify your interests.

Sixth, be ready to bounce back as life is full of lumps and bumps (my lump was cancerous). Try to take setbacks in stride and adapt. Two weeks after winning a senior men's tennis event, I developed a severely painful tendonitis known as *tennis elbow* that lasted 1 year before it was surgically repaired. In the meantime, I learned how play and compete left-handed. Resiliency is a good thing.

Seventh, cherish family and friends. Life would be much less meaningful if we were not connected to one another. Standing alone is not an expression of strength. Sharing our joys and our sorrows is a wonderful part of life. The time and energy required to solidify relationships is the best investment one can make.

* Muhammad Ali

Eighth, take advantage of nature and God's incredible playground. Enjoy the beauty of the flowers, mountains, rivers, rain, butterflies, a snow flurry, and the color of the deep green grass when Winter turns to Spring. Through our eyes, we can witness an endless number of stunning miracles that should never be overlooked or taken for granted.

Ninth, redefine and strengthen your value system. Establish a high standard of integrity and try to do what is right regardless of the circumstances. To err is human. Learn to apologize.

Lastly, tell those close to you that you love them. You will never regret having expressed these feelings, for tomorrow, this option may not exist. Life is not a destination, but rather a journey. I suspect that the "winner" is not the one with the most wealth, power, or prestige, but rather the one who most enjoyed the allotted time, doing his or her best along the way.

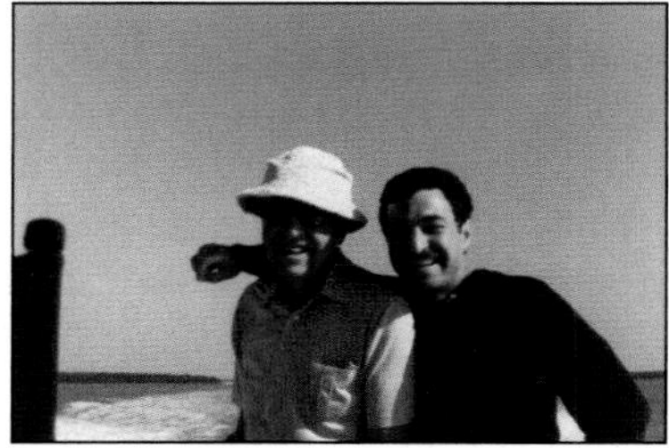

Epilogue

This short book started off as an urgent message—a legacy of sorts—that I needed to write for my children. It was intended to analyze the ingredients of Achievement, something that I understood, which might help to enrich each of their lives. However, as I recovered from my cancer surgery, the content written by a loving father began to change. I included other life topics as my own outlook about life was being transformed. When I was invited to give the Innovator's Award Lecture to the American Society of Cataract and Refractive Surgery in 2009, I questioned whether there might be anything in these pages that could also prove worthwhile to my colleagues. After all, I had invested 3 decades teaching surgeons on six continents how to manage challenging cases, and I would consider myself as challenging a case as it gets!

The second edition was published a full decade after the first. During this interval, my children grew up, I remarried, and nine exquisite grandchildren came into my life. According to my first wife, Barbara, I have mellowed. According to my current wife, Debbie, Barbara deserved a medal! I am still learning, still making mistakes, and always trying to be a better person. All in all, I feel very lucky. I love my job, I adore my family, I am in love, and I believe every day is a blessing. We get out of life what we put into it, and until I drop, I plan on going full speed ahead!

I hope that the mission of writing this book for my children has been accomplished. I also hope that I have not wasted anybody's precious time and that there is something in these pages that will make the reader's life a little more focused, a little more organized, and a little more enjoyable.

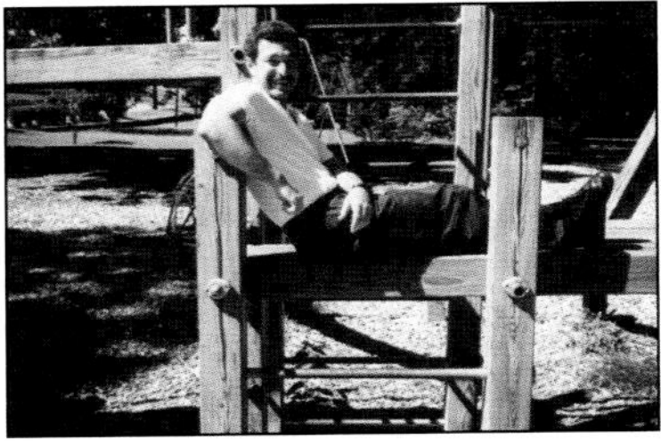

Acknowledgments

The second edition was an arduous project! Thanks to Linda Harris and Tonya Ragle for their extraordinary help with the manuscript and the photographs. Thanks to Peter Slack, President of The Wyanoke Group, for deciding to publish this book.

This was a lonely project! Thanks to my children and grandchildren for their unwavering love and support. Barbara helped me with the first edition, and Debbie's companionship was invaluable during this second edition. I worked into the morning hours many nights, yet I tried not to fall asleep before thanking the good Lord in my prayers. As I turn 70 years of age with most of my life behind me, I am grateful for the opportunity to share some of the lessons that have not only helped me in my quest for Achievement and Balance, but also in seeking and finally finding the elusive sense of Contentment—the Real ABCs.

Robert H. Osher, MD

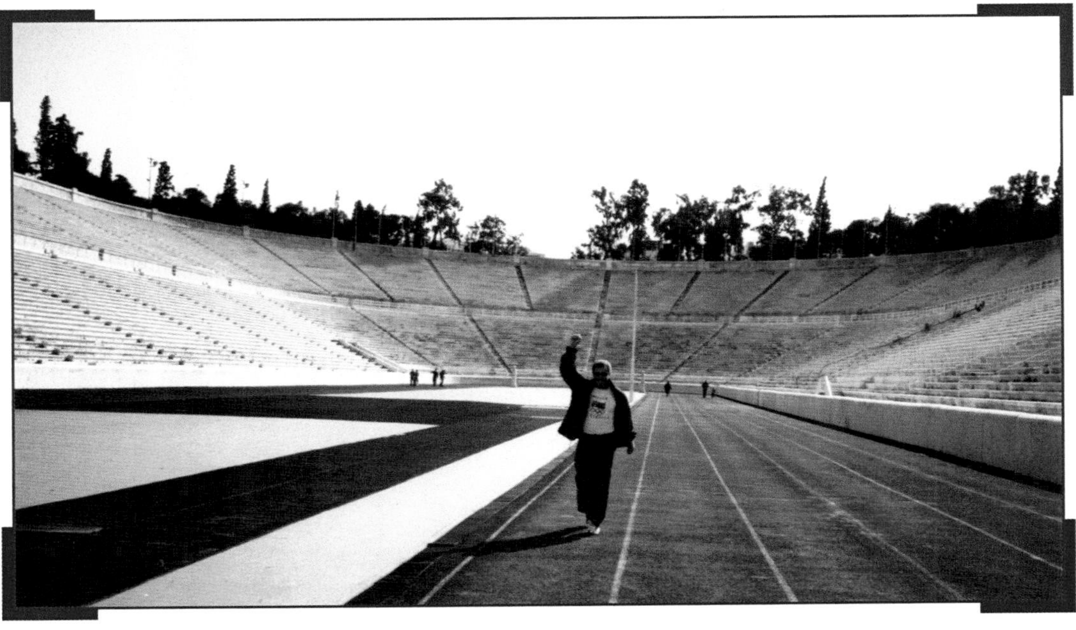